Recharge Your Body and Mind with Amazing Amino Acids

"I have known Dr. Dan Smith professionally for the past 20 years. As a clinical nutritionist, I've collaborated with Dr. Dan on hundreds of nutritional programs for the patients we have worked with together. I have always been impressed with Dr. Dan's intelligence, insights, and his ability to see the big picture. Dan has helped thousands of patients with his chiropractic care and in more recent days with his knowledge and use of amino acids. Early on Dr. Dan recognized the tremendous healing potential present in amino acids. As a visionary entrepreneur, Dr. Dan has made amino acid therapy available to the mainstream population with great success. This book, Recharge Your Body and Mind with Amazing Amino Acids, will help people to understand and utilize the powerful and potent benefits present in amino acids."

-TIM KUSS, CCN

"Amino acids are essential to our health and wellbeing. However, due to dietary deficiency, or poor ability to absorb or assimilate them, many people remain deficient—and end up suffering from fatigue, mood swings, or other mental or physical conditions. That's why I prescribe them to my patients on a regular basis. Dr. Dan Smith has researched this area thoroughly and created high quality, broad spectrum amino acids that boost both mental and physical health."

-HYLA CASS, MD, 8 WEEKS TO VIBRANT HEALTH

"I met Dr. Smith one afternoon at a conference in San Francisco, and we didn't stop talking about amino acids until late that evening. He was excited over his discoveries of the clinical potential of free-form amino acid therapy. I was pleased to find a person with a mind that grasped the implications of the therapy. Biochemists know about the role of amino acids as building blocks for proteins, etc., and nutritionists understand the importance of dietary protein intake. But it is the complex physiology of maldigestion and increased utilization in patients with degenerative disease that must be grasped to see why they may have normal protein intake and still be in a downward spiral of organ reserve loss because of insufficient blood amino acid supply. Use of free-form amino acids can be a key to reversing that spiral, and Dr. Smith had reams of evidence that real people for whom the usual medical interventions had failed responded beautifully to the practical application of amino acid formulas. So our meeting led to a rare merging of theory (me) and practicality (him) that was simply supposed to happen. His book can help you to see the outcome in terms of improving your health."

-RICHARD S. LORD, CHIEF SCIENCE OFFICER, METAMETRIX CLINICAL LABORATORY

Recharge Your Body & Mind with
AMAZING
AMINO ACIDS

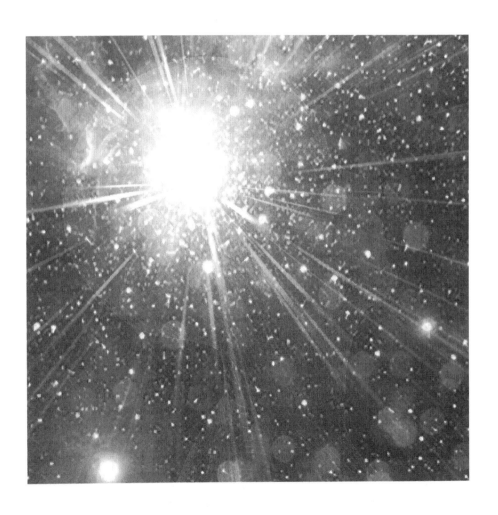

Dr. Daniel S. Smith, D.C.

Recharge Your Body and Mind with Amazing Amino Acids

By Dr. Daniel S. Smith, D.C.

Published by
Daniel S. Smith
Truckee, CA 96162

ISBN: 1478200146
ISBN 13: 9781478200147

Dedication

I would like to graciously dedicate this book to Robert Erdmann, Ph.D., and his wife Marie, both of whom passed on in 2006 and 2011, respectively. I remain dedicated to the vision Dr. Erdmann shared from decades of his research on the amazing benefits of broad-spectrum free-form amino acids for mental and physical health.

I believe his book, The Amino Revolution, lives on as his spirit soars. His wife, Marie, shared her enthusiasm and passion to continue this body of work and to share it with the world, as did her husband.

Dr. Daniel S. Smith, D.C.
January 12, 2014

Acknowledgments

Deepest thanks to those who helped make this book possible including Robert Erdmann, Ph.D., Don Tyson, Richard S. Lord, Ph.D., Hyla Cass, M.D., Judy Chang, Ph.D., Vanita Gibbs, Ph.D., Susan T. Sutton, R.N., Thad Mauney, Ph.D., Preston Wright, Ph.D., Caroline Wadlin, M.D., Carol Banyas, M.D., Ph.D., Teresa Kolpak, Tim Kuss, C.C.N., Susan Horst, David Moeglein, Diane Moeglein, and Cindy Leonard.

To the wonderful team at the E Learning Café, Incline Village, Nevada, thank you; with special thanks to Katherine Kelly, Ph.D., founder of the E Learning Café.

Special thanks to Pastor Wayne Hoag of the Sierra Bible Church in Truckee, CA., and the SBC-Men's support network; all who bring me strength and the passion of faith and fellowship to my life.

I am forever indebted to the town of Truckee, CA, and the passion this community shares to go out on a limb to bring healthy, safe food services to over 4,000 students at the Tahoe Truckee Unified School District and the opportunity to be involved in their pursuits.

Finally, a salute to the amazing amino acids and their counterpart: micronutrients; and to all nutrients that make us a healthier human race. I look forward to celebrating the day that this vision for mental/physical health would be embraced by the healthcare system worldwide—that the integration of healthy lifestyle, healthy, safe, fresh, affordable and accessible food combined with micronutrient solutions will be viewed as an essential component to OPTIMAL HEALTH.

Preface

The most common approach to improved nutrition, besides improving the diet, is to purchase specific nutritional products such as a multivitamin/mineral or an essential fatty acid supplement such as omega-3 fish oil. There is also a new movement to purchase a high-quality probiotic for gastrointestinal health. Given our bodies' needs for these essential nutrients to restore and maintain health, these are all actually good choices as a starting point.

However, what I have observed over a 25-year career as a practicing health care professional is that most individuals taking these expensive nutritional supplements, for the most part, still have the chronic ailments that brought them to take the supplements in the first place. They are approaching nutrition and health one piece of the puzzle at a time, quite possibly lacking key knowledge about how to integrate optimum nutrition into their lifestyles. Time and again I've seen patients spending money on medications or supplements without completely reclaiming their health or discovering how to truly be recharged.

In the early 2000s I began introducing my patients to free-form amino acids as an adjunct to chiropractic care—as a type of metabolic tune up. I first started using single, high doses of amino acids, such as tryptophan for mood and sleep disorders, tyrosine for a short memory problems and depression, and GABA for anxiety disorders. These are a few of the classic approaches to individual ailments with the use of amino acid therapy.

During my quest to find the perfect "metabolic tune up" for my patients, I read the book, *The Amino Revolution,* written by Robert Erdmann, Ph.D., in 1989. I had learned from a colleague that this was one of the most important books ever written on the subject of free-form amino acids. Dr. Erdmann wrote extensively on an amino acid formula that he called "the complete blend." It is here that I realized a brilliant concept had been overlooked by the health care industry. This simple concept, a whole and complete amino acid supplement, allows an individual's body and mind to "pick and choose" the needed amino acids as opposed to a health practitioner making an educated guess, using a "symptoms-only" approach, which often misses the big picture of the complex system of your total health.

This nutritional approach to health—amino nutrients—provides the synergy necessary for wellness and longevity. Amino acids are in fact the missing puzzle piece that brings all the nutrients to optimum performance.

According to Robert Lue, Ph.D., of Harvard University, "We have over 70 trillion living cells in our body." These cells range from heart cells, bone cells, brain cells, pancreas cells, gastrointestinal cells and so on. "In each of these trillions of cells there are tens of thousands of enzymatic chemical actions occurring every second," he explains. Think about that! These are astronomical numbers. The essential needs of fuelling these cells every second and the fuel for these enzymes are ALL found in amino acids. Amino acids demonstrate the beauty and miracle of the body and the universal intelligence that allows all this to happen in an order that maintains our human health.

Maintaining our health is more important than ever as we endeavour to live longer in toxic environments with fewer natural nutrients contributing to our longevity. Today society as a whole is clamouring for more than a simple fix; they are seeking a total solution.

As a healthcare provider, I am devoted to unlock these puzzle pieces for the general public, the intricate nutrient approach to total wellness, beginning with the nutrient powerhouse: amino acids. As building blocks they perfectly embody where we should all begin our personal wellness journeys; journeys that I personally believe also include linking food, family, health professionals and communities to the farm.

We've all gazed at rainbows, Mother Nature's full spectrum of color, shimmering in the sky. In doing so we are reminded of beauty, hope and new beginnings. We marvel at the miniature rainbows cast by prisms. No matter your favorite color, it is there within, enhanced by the whole.

This is the concept I specifically endorse in amino acid therapy. One amino acid may help with a particular problem, but with the presence of all, a broad spectrum of amino acids, its effectiveness is enhanced.

Striving for a small footprint with maximum return,

Dr. Dan

Table of Contents

CHAPTER 1

Do You Need Amino Acid Supplements?

According to the leading experts (specialists using amino acids as a therapy), there are individuals who require broad-spectrum amino acid supplementation more than others.

They are:

- Those on or who have been on prescription medications
- Those recovering from surgery
- Those who have any gastrointestinal disorders
- Those with a family history of degenerative diseases (i.e., heart disease, atherosclerosis, diabetes, cancer)

- Those with any genetic or enzymatic deficits that interfere with normal protein synthesis and metabolism

However, there are other health problems also associated with deficiencies and unbalanced amino acids. An imbalance in amino acids in the body can be caused by many things including strenuous exercise, aging, drug use, certain medications, infections, vitamin B or C deficiency, or even a lack of varied protein sources. Taking the quiz on the following page may help you determine if you are also a good candidate for amino acid supplementation.

Amino Acid Health Quiz

1. Do you experience fatigue upon arising in the morning?
2. Do you experience chronic emotional and/or physical pain?
3. Do you experience hypoglycemia symptoms?
4. Do you experience moodiness?
5. Do you experience ADD, depression, anxiety, panic attacks, sleeplessness, or fibromyalgia?
6. Do you have any chemical addictions?
7. Are you recovering from an injury?
8. Do you have a difficult time consuming enough protein at three meals per day?
9. Do you have food or other allergies/eating disorders?
10. Are you interested in supplements for well-being and anti-aging?
11. Are you a sports enthusiast/body builder?
12. Do you need additional support in your body's detoxification process due to environmental chemicals?

13. Have you had an illness and/or stress that have strained your body's resources?

14. Would like to strengthen your body's overall vitality?

———*༄༄༄*———

How did you do? The odds are that you not only answered yes once, but possibly several times. Is it really that easy to determine your need for amino acid supplementation? Yes! Each of the chapters in this book is designed to assist you in discovering for yourself how your body and your quality of life will benefit from the guided use of amino acid supplementation.

What are amino acids?

Amino acids are the essential building blocks of protein and for the basis of life itself. They are the raw materials for the growth and reproduction of every cell in the body and are present throughout the body. Amino acids are the materials that build the neurotransmitters in your brain, digestive enzymes and the enzymes that work in all metabolic pathways, the immune system and even stem cells. Every bone, organ, muscle, and almost all hormones are made from the combinations of amino acids with the help of vitamins, minerals and other cofactors.

Amino acid forms (D) and (L)

Amino acids are constructed from a combination of carbon, hydrogen, oxygen, nitrogen and in some cases sulfur. Every amino acid except glycine, the smallest of them, comes in two forms, a "left handed" (l) and a "right-handed" (d) form. These two forms contain the same elements, in precisely the same quantities and in the same sequence, but, they are the mirror image of each other.

The body is constructed almost completely from the (l) forms of amino acids. However, small amounts of the (d) forms occur naturally and some have therapeutic value. As we will see later, this is true for the (d) form of phenylalanine, which is a particularly valuable asset in treating pain.

For the sake of simplicity, all amino acids mentioned throughout the text are written without the (l) in front. However, when a (d) form is discussed, it is specified. For example, when you read about l-tryptophan, it will be written simply as tryptophan.

Note: In *Recharge Your Body and Mind with Amazing Amino Acids*, the amino acids recommended will always be broad-spectrum, free form, and pharmaceutical grade with essential cofactors; a "complete blend."

Is there any other kind? Yes. You will find amino acids in several different forms for consumer use. Some are sold as single amino acids, such as a bottle of tryptophan only. Broad-spectrum refers to the complete range of the 22 amino acids rather than single amino acids.

Some supplements provide amino acids bound in protein rather than free form. Why use free form? When amino acids are in their free form state, separated from the long protein molecule chain, the body doesn't need the intestinal tract to break them down; they are predigested. That means that they pass quickly through the intestinal wall and into the bloodstream.

There are other forms of amino acids that are not as bioavailable as free form, meaning they require digestion, thus taking longer to be available as building blocks, as well as losing mass in the digestive process. For example: You might not get the same results taking a protein powder. Doesn't that product contain amino acids? Yes. Is that the best supplement to give you a large amount of usable end products, without loss due to digestion? No.

What do we mean by a "complete blend?" A complete blend is the entire spectrum, the broad-spectrum of free form amino acids (10 essential and 12 nonessential), containing the necessary cofactors well-known for neurotransmitter synthesis in the brain and nervous system.

What if you find a product that has all of the amino acids without any of the cofactors? That's like trying to build a house without any builders. You might have great building supplies (the amino acids), but the jobs they need to perform will not get done without the cofactors; they are essential! Without these specific known cofactors the amino acid would not synthesize into the neurotransmitter. For example: tryptophan without B-6 would not become serotonin. Serotonin is a key neurotransmitter in the nervous center that helps maintain good mood.

An ideal complete blend should contain at least:

- alanine
- arginine
- asparagine
- aspartic acid
- cysteine
- GABA
- glutamine
- glutamic acid
- glycine
- histidine

- isoleucine
- leucine
- lysine
- methionine
- phenylalanine
- proline
- serine
- taurine
- threonine
- tryptophan
- tyrosine
- valine
- essential cofactors such as vitamin B, calcium, magnesium

To summarize: Throughout the book when the phrase "the complete blend" is mentioned, it is ALWAYS in direct reference to a broad-spectrum, free-form amino acid supplement with all of the amino acids and essential cofactors.

How important are amino acids for optimal brain health? Optimal brain health is critical for living healthier as we live longer. Modern science is making dramatic new discoveries about the health of the brain and the nervous system. These breakthroughs include discovering how naturally occurring chemicals renew and repair the brain and the nervous system. They are especially important because of our increased lifespan. We are accustomed to the terms "meno-pause" and "andro-pause." A new concept has been coined "cerebral-pause," which has to do with maintaining the health of the brain and the nervous system, the core systems of our body. The earlier in life preventative measures are taken to protect these vital systems, the greater our chances are for cognitive health as we age.

Our mental and emotional wellbeing is another vital area that amino acids are required for functioning properly. Communications within the brain and the nervous system occur through chemical "languages." Neurotransmitters are used in these languages to transmit messages from one neuron or nerve cell, to a specific organ such as a muscle or gland. Neurotransmitters are powerful chemicals that influence numerous physical and behavioral processes, including cognitive and mental performance, emotional states, and pain response.

What all that means is that every system in your body requires amino acids to function properly, from bones and organs to your digestive tract to your brain/nervous system and even your emotional wellbeing. These are some very powerful little nutrients—the amazing amino acids.

Throughout this book you will learn how to take amino acids for many different health concerns as well as how to maximize the effects of amino acids when you ingest them. You will learn about safety and precautions and the difference in dosages: maintenance dose, therapeutic effect dose, and an intensive, athletic performance training dose. You will also learn how much and when to take amino acids based on my findings over the years in private practice and from reports I receive from other health care professionals. However, because we are all unique individuals, you may need to modify the amount that you take as well as when to take amino acids.

Individual Amino Acids

A question I often hear is: what is the difference between taking single doses of amino acids and a complete blend of them? Certain individual amino acids can be successful in treating very specific symptoms. For example, the amino acid taurine can be critical in the prevention of seizures. Studies have shown that taurine provides aid for defects in nerve blood flow, motor nerve conductivity velocity and nerve sensory thresholds.

Certainly, when dealing with certain chronic and acute conditions in my private practice, I may combine single, high doses of amino acids with other micronutrients to establish immediate reduction in symptoms. However, I have found that leaning toward integration of a complete blend into a patient's diet offers in most cases a successful outcome to the widest array of symptoms and patients. Oftentimes illness causes a chain reaction of deficiencies where one symptom can be addressed with an individual amino acid but the stress of the illness itself on the overall system may need a complete blend of amino acids to assist in the necessary repairs towards optimal health.

Amino acids are integral to optimal health!

CHAPTER 2

What Are Amino Acids? Why Are They So Important to Your Health?

I have had the opportunity to read hundreds of research papers about free form amino acids and their role in mental and physical health. I have been privileged to interview, consult and even lecture with some of the top authorities in the world about free form amino acids and the role they play in our physical and mental health. Yet, even over a 20-year span of learning about these amazing amino acids with their potential for healing many types of symptoms and conditions, we are still just scratching the surface of the mystery of their origins, their potential, and the role they play in the health care industry today.

My personal story about amino acids is related to my 25-year career as a chiropractor in a small town in northern California. In the early 2000s I began having premonitions that a new model or a new approach to treating chronic neurological and behavioral disorders was emerging. I was not sure what this meant at the time. But I would jokingly share with friends and colleagues that someday, someone was going to discover a way to give a "virtual" chiropractic adjustment. Traditionally, our profession's philosophy is that by correcting spinal misalignments and relieving nerve pressure with a specific hands-on chiropractic adjustment to the misaligned vertebrae, you can relieve pain, and balance the brain and central nervous system by restoring clear communication between the body and the brain. This concept of balancing the nervous system from a chiropractic adjustment allows our natural innate intelligence to restore optimal function and health in each individual. I have always appreciated this philosophy for restoring health as naturally as possible. I have witnessed thousands of healings take place using spinal adjusting in my offices.

However, I wanted to help empower patients as well as the healthcare professional with tools that the patient could integrate into their lifestyle in between office visits, to maintain their progress or to enhance their care affordably. This idea of a "virtual" chiropractic adjustment followed me for several years. For example: I practiced yoga and considered developing a new chiropractic yoga model where a patient could be trained to keep a healthy, aligned spine. I could not relinquish the idea that the only way to receive the true benefits of a chiropractic adjustment is with a doctor's hands on the patient.

Then, in 2003, when I began reading *The Amino Revolution*, by Robert Erdmann, Ph.D., I knew there existed a different way to help and empower people to have better, sustainable health. I was inspired to truly explore the idea of a virtual tune-up.

It was a warm summer day. I had the afternoon off work and decided to lie out by the pool to relax and read. I was processing the section of Dr. Erdmann's book in which he describes amino acids and their role in the brain and central nervous system. He explained how amino acids are the building blocks for all the neurotransmitters in the brain and nervous system. He detailed how the neurotransmitters work to communicate messages from the brain to the body. He then described how these amino acids are the precursors to more than fifty neurotransmitters in the brain and nervous system, and that he had developed a possible nutritional formula with all the amino acids grouped together in one product, a complete blend.

At that moment in time, bells went off in my head. This was what I had been looking for—a way to balance the brain and nervous system. If I could give my patients a complete blend, they would in fact be receiving the first "virtual" chiropractic adjustment.

I went to work immediately. I hired two seasoned authors and authorities in the field of amino acid therapy. We added the well-known cofactors that are essential for neurotransmitter synthesis in the brain. We pursued the highest-quality ingredients. Eighteen months later we had developed a formula with a 30-year research pedigree behind it, in a modern composition.

I chose not to offer the product in the marketplace for the first six months as I wanted to use it in my private practice to really wrap my arms around its potential and its limitations with several types of patients and illnesses. What I found was an instant empowering impact on patients and a virtually untapped resource for wellness—all in a blend of amazing amino acids. To this day, after years of research, I still get excited about their unlimited potential to recharge the mind and body. The complete blend is truly proving itself universal to enhance patients' health and wellbeing as prescribed by integrative health care practitioners around the world.

That is just a quick summary of my journey into amino acids. Now, I would like to walk you through the intricate marvel of how amino acids work.

What are amino acids and how do they work?

Proteins comprise 75% of the dry weight of the human body (1). All proteins are composed of amino acids, the building blocks of life. Amino acids, alone or in combination with fatty acids, minerals and vitamins, are used by the body to build and repair cells including muscles, skin, hair, nails, bones, organs and glands. Such proteins are classified as *structural proteins.*

In addition, amino acids are the essential elements used to make metabolic and digestive enzymes; neurotransmitters, critical for brain and nerve function; hormones, produced by the thyroid, pituitary, ovaries, testes, pancreas, kidneys, adrenals, and other carrier and messenger cells. These are the *functional proteins.*

Scientists have isolated 22 amino acids our bodies use constantly, 10 of which are considered *essential* in the human diet. An *essential* amino acid is one that cannot be produced from other amino acids within the body and therefore must be obtained from dietary or supplemental sources. The *nonessential* amino acids are also required for healthy life, but can be provided either by dietary sources or by conversion from one of the essential amino acids. However, the conversion requires that the essential amino acid be adequately supplied, and that the conversion enzymes and cofactors are also adequate. If there is an impairment of the conversion process, a nonessential amino acid may become essential for healthy life under those special conditions, so it is called conditionally essential.

When we encounter disease, nutritional problems, or environmental toxins those conditionally essential amino acids can become very important. For this reason supplementation with nonessential amino acids is recommended. The 10 essential amino acids combined with the 12 nonessential amino acids meet the daily demands for our mental and physical health.

There are an estimated 100,000+ proteins found in the human body. Structural proteins build and renew every cell, organ, and system in your body. Functional proteins, including enzymes, carry out the metabolic functions of life itself. They are all made from combinations of essential and nonessential amino acids.

Supplementing a diet with amino acids, combined with healthy eating and adequate water intake, provides the nutritional support needed to maintain metabolic balance, build muscle, and repair damaged cells. *See Appendix D: 4.31 and 4.32.* They improve and stabilize mood, support and protect nerve function, balance your immune system, aid chronic fatigue, keep your heart healthy and more. Unlike amino acids derived from food sources, free-form, pharmaceutical-grade amino acids require no digestion. Absorption is rapid and complete.

The value of using a complete amino acid supplement ensures all of the amino acids are available when they are needed. When you experience emotional or physical stress, including injury, inflammation or infection, your body requires an increased supply of amino acids to support, defend and repair your body. Having these nutrients readily available in a form requiring no digestion for assimilation provides broad based amino acid nutrients to prevent or improve conditions such as heart disease, diabetes, hypoglycemia, depression, and more.

In respect to mood disorders, substance abuse and chemical dependency, many individuals find a combination of single, high dose, free-form amino acid supplement therapy, combined with a complete blend is the best combination for their recovery and healing. For more specific information, contact your integrative healthcare professional.

Evidence-Based Approach

Amino acids are the most gravely misunderstood of the essential nutrients required for healthy infants, children, adults and senior citizens. An abundance of scientific and clinical evidence has been published showing the usefulness and safety of amino acid supplementation in a variety of life situations. The references cited at the end of this book will give you access to some of the abundant evidence of their functions and benefits.

A complete blend of essential and nonessential free-form amino acids is suitable for pregnant and nursing women,[2] seniors needing extra nutritional support,[3-4] and athletes following intense physical exercise.[5] Another common use for the blend is to increase the benefits of fitness training and body building in young and old when taken just prior and after a workout.[6-7] A complete blend is also recommended to recover from eating disorders,[8] to recover from acute or chronic infectious disease or inflammation,[9-10] or to help control mood, especially depression or anger.[11]

In summary, amino acids are the building blocks for ALL protein structures. They also strengthen your bones because the mineral in your bones is held together by a tight matrix of collagen, a protein. Amino acids build strong nails, hair and provide healthy skin. They are also the precursors, the building blocks, to ALL the enzymes in your body. These thousands of enzymes make the vital processes in your body work: building the body structures, processing food into energy, and breaking down toxins and waste for removal. Two other important jobs amino acids have are to strengthen your immune system as well as to construct and synthesize more than fifty neurotransmitters in your brain and central nervous system.

Amino Acids and Aging

As we age, nutritional needs may actually increase, yet appetite may decrease, [12] so that we need more but get less. Amino acids have been found to be lower in both blood and muscle of aged humans.[13] Amino acid supplementation has shown exciting potential to restore and maintain the health of aging men and women, to improve muscle mass, protect from heart damage, increase muscle strength, improve insulin sensitivity and more.[14-16]

We are all concerned about the seemingly inevitable increases in heart disease, adult onset diabetes, sarcopenia (muscle wasting associated with aging), age-related depression and loss of memory. Research over the past few years has shown daily supplementation of essential amino acids improves muscle mass with or without exercise,[17] as well as reducing insulin resistance,[18] a common complication of aging and a precursor to the development of Type II adult onset diabetes.

Amino acid supplementation protects the brain and heart and increases muscle mitochondria while reducing muscle fibrosis (inactive fibrous tissue replacing healthy muscle). [19] Mitochondria are the powerhouses of all of our cells, and aging is associated with decreased mitochondria in muscle and brain. Restoring essential mitochondria is an important part of any anti-aging program.

Amino acids also increase the production of essential enzymes, which enhance and protect muscles, including the heart, and the brain. We often think of enzymes in terms of digestion, and amino acids do support healthy digestion, but every metabolic change throughout the body and brain is actually controlled and modified by enzymes. [20-21]

We are all aware that exercise is important for both body and brain. Significant daily exercise reduces blood pressure, heart disease, insulin resistance, obesity, osteoporosis and even depression. [22-24] When exercising is difficult due to fatigue, weakness, or muscle insufficiency, amino acids have been shown to improve exercise capacity. [25-26]

Inactivity, often accompanying aging and illness, alters the body's ability to utilize protein. Free-form amino acid supplementation, which requires no digestion, shows potential to reverse this condition, as well as the muscle wasting caused by corticosteroid medications. [27] This, in turn, may allow one to begin a regular program of physical activity, an important component for overall health and longevity.

A complete blend of amino acids addresses issues of aging by providing not just a complement of essential amino acids, but also several conditionally essential amino acids. These include carnitine to improve fat burning, cognitive function and heart function, [28-29] and taurine, a membrane stabilizer, anti-oxidant, and calcium stabilizer, as well as a key component of the functioning muscle, heart, brain and eye. [30-33] In addition taurine, along with other amino acids, has shown the benefit of learning and memory retention and is necessary for a functioning immune system. [34-37]

As you can see, each amino acid is a nutrient powerhouse, synergistically supporting health as well as healthy aging.

What is a nutrient?

You might be wondering at this point, what exactly is a nutrient, a "micronutrient" or a "macronutrient?"

A nutrient is a substance that provides nourishment essential for growth and the maintenance of life. To function, the human body must have nutrients.

The nutrients known to be essential for human beings are:

- Proteins
- Carbohydrates
- Fats and Oils
- Minerals
- Vitamins
- Water

Proteins, carbohydrates, fats and oils are needed in large quantities daily, and are therefore classified as macronutrients.

Micronutrients are nutrients required by humans and other living things throughout life in small to microscopic quantities. These orchestrate a whole range of physiological functions. They include amino acids, essential fatty acids, vitamins and minerals. Because the quantities of these micronutrients are so small, deficiencies in the foods we serve might be overlooked, and nutritional supplements are very helpful in assuring that we get an adequate supply of them.

Optimal nutrition requires approximately forty essential nutrients, including: amino acids, vitamins, minerals, and essential fatty acids.

What happens when we fall short of that optimal nutrition in our daily intake? A world renown biochemist, Bruce Ames, Ph.D., stated that, "…when one input in the metabolic network is inadequate, repercussions are felt on a large number of systems and can lead to…disease." Yet, "…an optimum intake of micronutrients and metabolites, which varies with age and genetic constitution, would tune up metabolism and give a marked increase in health...at little cost." (38)

Clearly, optimal health requires the full spectrum of nutrients. And, when one puzzle piece or one nutrient is missing, it can be felt throughout all the body processes. So, how important are amino acids in the nutrient puzzle?

According to a well-known expert in the field, Eric Braverman, M.D., Ph.D., author of *The Healing Ingredients Within*, "...we have harvested the vitamins and minerals as healing nutrients, and are just beginning to harvest the amino acids, which are even more important." (39) The importance of amino acids cannot be stressed enough!

A hidden amino acid deficiency can lead to multiple physical and emotional difficulties and a variety of symptoms including:

- hypoglycemia/moodiness
- low serotonin conditions resulting in depression, anxiety, panic, insomnia and fibromyalgia
- low endorphin conditions resulting in chronic physical and emotional pain

However, a broad spectrum free-form blend, or what I call *a complete blend*, provides benefits without needing to measure exactly which amino acids are deficient or why. To put it in another way: "A rising tide lifts all boats."

Most illnesses and/or stresses are likely to cause a chain reaction of nutritional deficiencies, straining enzyme and hormone production, protein synthesis, and the nervous system. This is where a complete blend can help restore what has been lost by this chain reaction, replenishing and strengthening the body's overall vitality.

The beauty of modern wellness is that this restorative effect can be provided safely and cost-effectively by using a complete blend, without always having to identify all specific imbalances.

The amino acid truly is a nutrient powerhouse!

CHAPTER 3

The Importance of Amino Acids, Probiotics and Gastrointestinal Function

According to the text, *Laboratory Evaluations for Integrative and Functional Medicine*, Lord, Brally, 2008, "proper gastrointestinal function, 'digestion,' is critical to adequate nutritional status and can impact all aspects of body function."

Approximately one-third of a person's daily caloric expenditure is required to drive the digestive, assimilative and immune functions while maintaining the gastrointestinal tract. [40] A large amount of the body's total lymphatic tissue is located in the gut and the gastrointestinal system is the only organ system of the body with its own independent lymphatic and nervous systems. The prime importance of the digestive system to overall health is indicated by the large number of total-body resources dedicated to it. [41]

Suffering from poor digestion upsets this balance and causes your body more harm than you can probably imagine. You can eat an excellent diet, with a full balance of vitamins, minerals, essential fatty acids and proteins, but unless the food is digested properly, your body simply won't be able to grow and repair itself as it should.

Stress, infection, poor dietary habits, environmental toxins and more can lead to digestive problems. Whatever the cause, the simple fact is that when your digestion doesn't work as it should, your cells are starved of the nutrients they need for healthy living. Toxins that cause oxidation and cell degeneration are allowed to build up. Growth and resistance to disease are reduced. Your skin gets blotchy, your body feels heavy and sluggish, and your emotions may become exaggerated and unstable.

Treating Gastrointestinal Disorders

Thus, good digestion is one of the first lines of defense for health and wellness. A complete blend ingested with a probiotic can have a synergistic impact on detoxifying and healing gastrointestinal disorders. Probiotic supplements provide the special bacteria our intestines need for healthy digestion. I personally prefer a probiotic that contains prebiotics—the special foods that probiotics need for optimal digestive life. Together they promote a healthy digestive environment. The probiotic and prebiotic supplements work as a good fertilizer would work to improve the soil in agriculture. Regular consumption of probiotics include enhanced immune function, improved colonic integrity, decreased incidence and duration of intestinal infections, downregulated allergic response and improved digestion and elimination processes. [42]

When working in tandem with probiotics, amino acids are actually one of nature's uncelebrated answers to gastrointestinal problems. Amino acids work to strengthen the immune system, detoxify unhealthy bacteria and tissue in the gut, and rebuild new gastrointestinal cells.

Amino Acid Absorption

Dr. Richard Lord has demonstrated that free-form amino acids enter the bloodstream approximately 20 minutes after ingestion. [42] The amino acid levels then remain mildly elevated for about sixty minutes after entering the bloodstream. [43] Research indicates that it is the rate of absorption and amount of time the free-form amino acids remain in the bloodstream that bring about such a positive impact on your health. (*See Appendix D: 4.31.*)

Once in the bloodstream, amino acids can help to reestablish normal digestive functions, strengthening the pancreas and stimulating the production of digestive acids and enzymes. [45] The pancreas produces over 15,000 enzymes. Amino acids are the building blocks for all of them. As they are produced, many of them flow from the pancreas to the small intestine as digestive enzymes that break down food for proper and healthy assimilation.

Additional actions to consider for improved gastrointestinal health:

- Include nutrient-dense whole foods such as greens, nuts and seeds in your diet.
- Add high-fiber ingredients to your diet.
- Increase intake of foods that contain omega 3 fatty acids such as wild salmon and walnuts.

- Increase your intake of saturated fats with extra virgin coconut oil.
- Avoid nutritional deficiencies by complementing nutrient dense foods with quality supplementation.
- Supplement your diet with quality digestive enzymes (typically found in raw foods but can be taken as a supplement).
- Stop eating two hours before bedtime.
- Chew your food thoroughly to aid digestion.
- Eat small meals throughout the day, rather than large, heavy meals.
- Drink plenty of water between meals.

Avoid foods that irritate the digestive system such as:

1. Alcohol
2. Caffeinated beverages such as coffee, tea, and soft drinks
3. Dairy products
4. Foods that contain gluten
5. Refined sugars and artificial sweeteners
6. Nitrites found in processed foods such as hot dogs, lunch meats and bacon
7. Monosodium glutamate (MSG) found in many foods as a flavor enhancer
8. Partially hydrogenated oils found in many processed baked goods and snack foods
9. Deep-fried food, fast food, and junk food

Good digestion starts with amazing amino acids!

CHAPTER 4

Mood Disorders Part One:
Depression and Apathy

Depression

The exact cause of depression is not proven. Many researchers believe it is caused by chemical changes in the brain. This may be due to genetic and or enzymatic deficits, or it can be triggered by serious life events. It is also likely to be a combination of these. Some types of depression run in families.

Some stressors that may lead to depression are:

- Substance abuse
- Chronic alcohol intake
- Sleeplessness
- Loss of any significant relationship
- Death of someone close to you
- Childhood neglect or abuse
- Loss of a career
- Gastrointestinal disorders such as celiac disease or gluten intolerance

The symptoms of depression can vary from irritability, agitation, fatigue, becoming withdrawn, a sense of worthlessness and more. Any of these symptoms can become almost unbearable. If you are experiencing these types of symptoms for more than two to three weeks you should make an appointment with your physician to seek help and guidance. Spiritual assistance can also be beneficial.

One common thread I observed in private practice with different depression situations is that the individual often begins to stop taking care of himself or herself, i.e., quits eating healthy foods, quits exercising, sleeps too little or too much, and quits taking necessary nutritional supplements. Unfortunately, this only exacerbates the depression. One component of that could be that unhealthy eating and skipping the supplements leads to low key amino acids in the body.

To understand how amino acid deficiency exacerbates depression, it is important to understand how the brain affects our emotional and mental health. The primary neurotransmitters that maintain healthy brain functions are serotonin, GABA, dopamine and norepinephrine. Kept in balance, these neurotransmitters aid mood, sleep and anxiety.

Serotonin and GABA have a calming and inhibitory effect on the brain and on your mood, whereas dopamine and norepinephrine have a stimulating and excitatory effect on the brain and on your mood. The balance of these four neurotransmitters is critical to experiencing life with passion, energy, focus, and zest. One way to attain that important balance is with a complete amino acid blend.

Some of the ways using a complete blend helps improve mood disorders include:

- Providing adequate supplies for the brain to replenish its reserves of amino acids
- Facilitating the formation of neurotransmitters and neuropeptide messenger molecules
- Providing the building blocks for the brain to restore its own enzyme levels
- Increasing your body's endorphins to decrease physical and emotional pain

The most common response I receive from patients taking a complete blend is, "I feel more centered." This comment still amazes me today. If a patient's primary symptom was that they felt apathetic and depressed, more often than not, after going on a complete blend and dietary change protocol, they would come back after seven to 14 days and share that they feel more centered, and the apathy and depression were gone or reduced. If a patient's main symptom was that they felt a lack of focus and had hyperactive tendencies, after going on a complete blend and dietary change protocol, more times than not, they would come back after seven to 14 days and share that they felt more centered, and that they had more focus and less anxiety.

It is important to note that individuals with certain risk factors may require medication to address their depression. Many individuals have been able to overcome the negative impact of these risk factors through therapy, nutrition, exercise and faith. Unfortunately, this is not always the case. If you find that managing your life with quality food, nutritional supplements and healthy lifestyle choices does not relieve your depression, it is likely you are a candidate for prescription medications to manage your depression. Even if this is the case, many find ingesting the amino acid complete blend is complementary to prescription medications.

Some risk factors to take into consideration include:

- Biological influences
- Psychosocial influences
- Childhood maltreatment
- Family and genetic factors
- Stressful life events

Something else to consider is that individuals with moderate levels of depression or greater usually have a history of some gastro-intestinal disorder. They may not even be overtly aware of the issue. This needs to be addressed early in any treatment regimen.

In regards to mood, some of the individual amino acids in a complete blend are particularly helpful. Tryptophan is the amino acid that is the building block or precursor for serotonin. Serotonin is a neurotransmitter responsible for maintaining a healthy mood. It also aids in sleep, decreases carbohydrate cravings, enhances emotional flexibility, gives us a positive outlook on life and supplies our sense of humor. Interestingly, tryptophan is an essential amino acid and is the most difficult amino acid to get from your diet on a regular basis.

The amino acid GABA is your body's natural tranquilizer and can be taken as a supplement to build GABA in your brain. As the main inhibitory neurotransmitter in the brain, GABA provides calmness, relaxation and stress tolerance. It is synthesized from glutamic acid with vitamin B6 as a cofactor. Supplemental free-form GABA does offer a quick surge of GABA to stabilize mood, but support for synthesis provides more lasting supply, which is certainly more optimal. The amino acid glutamine serves as a reserve from which glutamate and GABA can be synthesized.

The amino acids tyrosine and phenylalanine, along with vitamin B-6, are required for the synthesis of dopamine and norepinephrine. When your brain is not building the proper amounts of dopamine and/or norepinephrine, you can begin to feel depressed or apathetic, feel a lack focus, or suffer from attention deficit disorder. These chemicals enhance alertness, energy, mental focus, drive and enthusiasm.

As you can see, neurotransmitters are not only integral to our emotional and mental wellbeing, but they rely on the amazing amino acids to manage all their tasks.

Apathy

Apathy is a mood of indifference or lack of motivation and can be very problematic. Many times it is due to a chemical imbalance that results in a dopamine deficiency, resulting in a depressed state. The question is: how can you energize your brain's metabolism and fuel the brain with the amino acids needed to build the neurotransmitters that energize your brain? Can this be accomplished without having to go on prescription psychotropic medications?

According to author John McManamy, "apathy and depression are clearly related. A review article by Robert van Reekum, M.D., from the University of Toronto in the winter 2005 *Journal of Neuropsychiatry*, reports on studies that found both apathy and depression endemic in populations with neuropsychiatric diseases and brain damage. Few were just one or the other. Depression and apathy were a package deal." [46]

The real breakthrough for me in treating depression and mood disorders successfully was when I stopped using just specific amino acids to treat the symptoms. With the use of a complete blend and chelated vitamins and minerals, patients would report feeling "more centered." Note: Proper dosing and frequency are key factors in a successful outcome.

That is the breakthrough I want to share with you! I have personally observed that a complete blend balances the inhibitory and the excitatory neurotransmitters, evening out an individual's moods.

It is also clear that amino acids have other very significant jobs to do outside of the brain and central nervous system, such as assisting in stabilizing your blood sugar, providing the building blocks for insulin, strengthening the immune system and increasing the amount of digestive enzymes. All these functions play a significant role in your body and your brain's holistic wellbeing. This is just another advantage of broad-spectrum amino acid choices.

The Importance of Protein in Combating Mood Disorders

Eating protein is key to maintaining brain health and preventing chemical imbalances in the brain. As I mentioned before, amino acids are the precursors for all the neurotransmitters in the brain and nervous system. When you are experiencing stress and/or life changes, it becomes even more important that you eat protein at each meal, as this is the fuel for maintaining these important chemicals in the brain. The optimal protein intake at each meal is approximately 20 grams. It is also important that you are choosing high quality animal protein (if you eat meat) and fresh, seasonal and local vegetables as often as possible.

Chicken, turkey, fish and lean meats are your best choices. I insist on grass-fed animal protein when I am purchasing meat for my home and try to find restaurants with this quality of food whenever I can.

High quality animal protein has more essential nutrients to naturally fuel your cells throughout your body. Avoid fueling your body and brain with animal protein that has had poor dietary intake standards, been raised in a stressful environment, been given hormones to speed growth, or been processed resulting in little nutritional value. Each of these unnatural processes leads to the poor health of the animal, which is passed onto you during ingestion.

Remember the key point here is to eat quality protein at breakfast, lunch and dinner. The protein is broken down in the stomach and gastrointestinal tract into amino acids, which enter your blood stream and support the chemicals in your brain that stabilize your mood, assist in your sleep, and maintain the proper nerve flow throughout your nervous system.

However, if you are depressed, attempting to take care of food choices often becomes almost impossible. This can lead to another component of depression: craving sweets. Chemical imbalances in the brain frequently result in individuals becoming addicted to sugar and carbohydrates, which, unfortunately, only amplify the depression. Thus it is so important to consider diet as well as supplementation when attempting to reduce or alleviate the symptoms of depression.

Mood balance begins with sufficient amino acid intake!

CHAPTER 5

Mood Disorders Part Two: Seasonal Affective Disorder, PMDD and Postpartum Depression

Seasonal Affective Disorder (SAD)

Many people dread the shortening of the days as winter approaches. They are susceptible to what we coin, "the winter blues." Short days and long nights of winter can be an annual descent into sadness and depression. Seasonal affective disorder (SAD) results from a neuro-hormonal imbalance that is linked to the amount of daylight and to the ticking of the body's biological clock. In the sun-belt states, where there is plenty of sunshine all year long, only 1% of the population has SAD, but in Washington and Alaska, the long winter nights affect up to 10% of the population.

Like depression, SAD appears to be a serotonin deficiency problem. If you have a history of "feeling blue" during the winter months, it is important to start a routine by mid-autumn to build your reserves with an amino acid supplement. It is best to begin taking a complete amino acid blend beginning in October. You can also choose to increase your intake if you are already on a program. However, by starting early in anticipation of the symptoms, this gives ample time for your body to gain momentum and, with good fortune, go through the season with passion and joy, instead of the dreaded blues.

Vitamin D and Seasonal Affective Disorder (SAD)

High doses of vitamin D during the winter months have also proven in several studies to be a very effective natural remedy for SAD, leading many health practitioners to believe that normal neurotransmitter function depends in part on adequate vitamin D synthesis. [47-48] Sunlight on the skin is an essential part of our natural way of synthesizing vitamin D, so of course with short dark days, plus heavy clothing, we make far less in winter and our reserves can be depleted. Vitamin D can be supported by eating foods like cod liver oil that contain high levels naturally, or by taking nutritional supplements. [49-51]

Even though wintertime sunlight in northern regions may not be intense enough for vitamin D synthesis, there is another benefit of sensible sun exposure. Sunlight influences another mood regulating hormone, melatonin.

Melatonin helps modulate your circadian (day/night) rhythms. Darkness triggering melatonin secretion by the pineal gland within your brain, brings you down gently at night for sleep. Sunlight shuts off melatonin production, bringing us up for daytime activity. If the day/night melatonin cycle is disrupted, insomnia, mood swings and food cravings may follow. Getting some sunlight early in the day can greatly help in restoring that cycle, which is why doctors recommend getting outdoors as a helpful remedy for jet lag.

Because of the influence of sunlight, melatonin levels and vitamin D levels tend to go in opposite directions. Most of us can sense the positive influence of sunlight in our own lives by the immediate lift we get from taking a walk outdoors on a beautiful sunny day. Of course there are many factors at work that brighten our mood in such cases, but sun exposure almost certainly is a critical part. Soaking in the warmth of the sun is one of the most relaxing activities we share with all living creatures; just watch a cat dozing in a beam of sunlight.

Premenstrual Dysphoric Disorder (PMDD)

When a woman experiences mood swings correlated with her monthly cycle that are so severe as to interfere with normal activities and relationships it might be classified as Premenstrual Dysphoric Disorder (PMDD). This condition includes symptoms of tension, irritability and depression greatly worsening before menstruation and much more severe than the better known premenstrual syndrome (PMS). Because PMDD is a significant medical condition, if you experience these symptoms please consider visiting a qualified health professional to get proper diagnosis and support.

The symptoms of PMDD include:

- Disinterest in daily activities and relationships
- Fatigue or low energy
- Feelings of sadness or hopelessness, possibly suicidal thoughts
- Feelings of tension or anxiety
- Feeling out of control
- Food cravings or binge eating
- Mood swings marked by periods of teariness
- Panic attacks
- Persistent irritability
- Physical symptoms such as bloating, breast tenderness, headaches, joint or muscle pain
- Sleeplessness
- Difficulty concentrating

These serve as a quick screening panel for PMDD. If five or more symptoms are occurring, including at least one mood symptom, PMDD can be suspected. A precise psychiatric diagnosis according to the DSM IV is a matter for professionals because it requires evaluation of the number of symptoms and scoring their severity and relationship to the menstrual cycle.

Even though there is not yet a generally accepted theory as to why a woman's menstrual cycle causes fluctuation in anxiety, tension, irritability and depression, it seems obvious that the neurotransmitters involved in mood regulation must be involved. Therefore, boosting the nutrients required by the brain for making these neurotransmitters seems logical and can be accomplished by ingesting a complete amino acid blend. In these situations it seems especially important to be sure to include the vitamin cofactors that enable the brain's enzymes to convert the free-form amino acids into the actual neurotransmitters. A classic example is vitamin B6, which helps make the calming neurotransmitter GABA.

For stubborn and/or deep, more intense biological imbalances, the optimal dosage is 9,400 mg (2,350 mg taken four times a day). Take a complete blend of the amino acids first thing in the morning, midmorning, mid-afternoon and before bedtime. These amino acids will enter your bloodstream within 20 minutes after ingestion, building serotonin in the brain, balancing your hormones, energizing your brain, calming your anxiety and giving you a new sense of life, called your "old self."

Other factors that increase the risk of PMDD or worsen the symptoms include any excessive use of alcohol, lack of exercise, obesity, and even drinking excessive amounts of coffee. So it would make sense to correct these as much as you can. Even a modest amount of exercise can make a big difference very quickly. Cutting coffee to minimum levels can avoid those edgy feelings that worsen anxiety and tension without providing any real boost in energy or focus.

Micronutrients and Pregnancy

Along with a well balanced diet, other nutritional factors are critically important to consider during pregnancy. Adequate nutritional support is imperative at every stage of a pregnancy, including meeting the body's daily micronutrient demands with good wholesome food, augmented with a complete blend, a vitamin/mineral, and omega 3 essential fatty acids.

Remember, you're eating for two. Thus, your nutritional choices during this time can have far-reaching repercussions. Recent observations in nutrition/lack of nutrition during pregnancy include:

1. Depletion of nutrient reserves throughout pregnancy can increase a woman's risk for maternal depression.
2. Women require more vitamins and minerals during pregnancy. Supplements can improve their nutritional and hemoglobin status.
3. Supplements also help improve and maintain functional immunity.
4. Many vitamins and minerals play important roles in gene regulation as well as in cellular metabolism and fetal growth.

Postpartum Depression (PPD)

The birth of a baby is normally a joyful event, but the accumulated stresses on the mother's body can be just too much. In fact, 30% to 75% of women encounter mood difficulties shortly after giving birth. Most recover their emotional balance quickly, but for some there are serious difficulties, including outright depression. Unfortunately, the mainstream approach to treating postpartum depression with psychotropic medications can be debilitating. Fortunately, there are other options! Health care professionals routinely share with me how effective they find recommending a complete blend of amino acids to new mothers experiencing postpartum depression.

The spectrum of postpartum psychiatric illness generally includes postpartum blues, postpartum depression (PPD) and postpartum psychosis. In addition, the postpartum period may be a time of increased risk for anxiety disorders such as panic disorder and obsessive-compulsive disorder.

Postpartum blues are characterized by mood (depressed or irritable), interpersonal hypersensitivity, and tearfulness. [52] They typically arise and resolve within 7 to 14 days following delivery.

As mentioned already, up to 70% of new mothers experience some level of sad and unstable moods, but most recover their emotional equilibrium fairly quickly.

Postpartum depression is defined as a major depressive episode starting within four weeks after delivery. Symptoms can include suffering from depressed mood for most of the day on most days, extreme sadness, mood swings, anxiety, sleeplessness, loss of appetite, irritability, and suicidal ideation. A 1996 review and analysis of 59 studies on the prevalence of PPD concluded that across many cultures 10% to 15% of women are affected, with an overall average of 13%. [53] That makes it a major public health problem. No improvement was evident a decade later when the US CDC surveyed women in 17 states and found a rate averaging 14% overall. [54]

The frequency of major depression shortly after childbirth is two to three times the rate among women in general (around 5% according to the CDC in 2006 to 2008)[55]. Similarly, the frequency of hospitalization for all psychiatric illnesses combined is higher in the first month after delivery than at any other time in a woman's life. The reasons for this are still unclear, although several theories have been proposed, including social, cultural, and biological factors. Among the facts known are that in the first three to four days after giving birth, estrogen levels drop a hundred to a thousand fold.

Recent studies at the University of Toronto have discovered that simultaneous with this estrogen reduction, levels of the enzyme monoamine oxidase A (MAO-A) increase dramatically throughout the brain within days after delivery. [56] This enzyme breaks down the neurotransmitters serotonin, dopamine and norepinephrine. As well as being responsible for transmitting signals between nerve cells, these neurotransmitters also influence our mood. If they are deficient, we initially feel sad and later have a high risk of becoming depressed.

Dietary supplements that are precursors to the monoamine neurotransmitter during the early postpartum period would be a way to help maintain sufficient levels of these neurotransmitters to maintain healthy mood. This would include the amino acids tryptophan and tyrosine, which the body can convert into the neurotransmitters serotonin, norepinephrine, and dopamine, respectively. These are included in a complete blend. Moreover, supplementation with a complete blend of amino acids is compatible with breast feeding, unlike some of the prescription psychotropic medications.

With a complete blend, the most common responses from women suffering with postpartum depression are reduced anxiety and panic as well as improved sleep and mood, with few or no side effects.

Amino acids are truly "rechargers" for the prevention and treatment of the blues!

CHAPTER 6

Anxiety

I did not intentionally set out to determine if a complete blend would aid in relieving anxiety disorders. I only knew that I had discovered amino acids are a powerful healing approach with patients, and that these amino acids are the building blocks to all the neurotransmitters in the brain and nervous system.

It is interesting the way nature works within us at various times in our lives. I had an emotionally challenging childhood due to many factors, including being a highly sensitive child. As a result, I experienced acute and chronic stressful situations leading to early child developmental anxiety issues, which I carried into my adult life. I chose to enter into psychotherapy at the young age of 26 rather than pay the price of living each day with an ongoing chronic anxiety disorder.

In my early studies about anxiety, I became aware of Dr. Elaine Aron's book, *The Highly Sensitive Person*. Her book offers some relevance as to why some individuals may experience childhood anxiety, whereas others do not. Here are a few comments from her book:

- "Your trait of being highly sensitive or having deep feelings is normal. It is found in 15 to 20% of the population, too many to be a disorder, but not enough to be well understood by the majority of those around you."

- "It is innate...this trait reflects a certain type of survival strategy, being observant before acting. The brains of highly sensitive persons actually work a little differently than others."

- "You are more aware than others of subtleties. This is mainly because your brain processes information and reflects on it more deeply. So even if you wear glasses, for example, you see more than others by noticing more."

- "Highly sensitive people are not overly sensitive or emotionally instable they are deep feeling individuals. Highly sensitive people are individuals that make fabulous artists, musicians, and healers. Their central nervous system literally has more sensory nerves as 'connectors' for the brain centers of emotions, music and art. As this attribute is validated in their developing years, it can do a lot for their self-esteem and development toward their true skills in life. If gone unnoticed it can lead to self-esteem disorders."

I participated in a long-term healing process in therapy to understand and heal the nature of my anxiety. I needed to talk it through and feel the hard feelings, develop myself (as a musician would practice all levels of the science, art and philosophy of music to become fully integrated) and through this process I had the opportunity to integrate the parts that were never developed in my childhood.

One critical discovery I found toward the end of my therapy was when I learned about amino acids along with other micronutrients and their value in maintaining an uplifted focus. So, as soon as I had formulated my version of a complete blend, I began taking it, along with a high-quality vitamin/mineral supplement. The combination of these essential nutrients offered me a remarkable sense of balance and focus.

Understanding anxiety will help you understand the impact amino acids can have on this particularly painful condition. Anxiety is a psychological state, characterized by physical, emotional, cognitive and behavioral components. Anxiety can be an intense emotion that is a displeasing feeling of fear and concern. It is actually considered a normal reaction to a stressor. But if the anxiousness becomes chronic, it is considered an anxiety disorder.

The symptoms of anxiety disorder are:

- Excessive worry
- Restlessness
- Irritability
- Fatigue

- Difficulty in concentration
- Muscle tension
- Sleeplessness

Recovery from anxiety disorders may require having someone you can trust to talk through all the levels of fear and concern. I recommend finding a good therapist or asking your church for support to assist you on your quest.

In some individuals, seasonal changes, dietary changes, stress and other factors can have a tendency to result in an exacerbation of symptoms. It is best to stick with a good diet, manage stress, exercise regularly and avoid the nuances that may retrigger anxiety in your life. If you find under unusually stressful conditions that conservative care is not enough to balance out the symptoms, you need to contact your healthcare professional for treatment recommendations.

My recommendation for the recovery of anxiety disorder is the integration of a complete blend into your daily dietary intake. Specifically for anxiety, I would recommend a therapeutic dose. *See Appendix A: How to Take Amino Acids.*

If you are on medications to manage anxiety, always discuss any changes you would like to make in your medications with your health care professional. Ultimately, you should be able to drop the medications as you balance your brain chemistry, stabilize your blood sugar, strengthen your immune system and heal your gastrointestinal tract.

After a six-to-twelve week period, you can begin to reduce your intake. However, if you are feeling anxious again you can return to the therapeutic dose at any time.

I found that developing a strong faith in God was essential for me, in recovering and healing my anxiety disorder. The fact is, we are all ultimately bound to the human condition, and we all ultimately die and leave our bodies. That's definitely something one can feel anxious or concerned about. Having a powerful faith in God allows us to understand that even the ultimate change, death, has a loving and comforting component to offer our lives.

Amino Acids and Anxiety

One of the primary reasons people choose to take a complete blend is that it calms their anxiety. The reason a complete blend works so well for anxiety disorder is fourfold:

- A complete blend fuels all the neurotransmitters in the brain and central nervous system. *See page 66: Amino Acid Nutrition Therapy Chart.*

- A complete blend helps to stabilize the blood sugar.

- A complete blend enters your blood stream within 20 minutes after ingestion. This rapid rate of entry has an immediate therapeutic effect. The strain anxiety unloads on your system causes the nutrients to be used up faster than normal. Yet the amino acids offer necessary energizing nutrients, rapidly coming to aid. *See Appendix D: 4.31, 4.32 and 4.2.*

- Anxiety causes the body to use up more nutrients than normal due to the stress and tension that build up. A complete blend immediately replaces the essential nutrients your body's demands. Without the added nutrients, the anxiety can become more amplified.

- People experiencing chronic anxiety disorder should also avoid stimulants like coffee and desensitizers like sugar, alcohol and nicotine to have a successful outcome. Further, it is critical to learn about the power of deep, prolonged sleep, which is covered in the next chapter, the power of sleep and how free-form amino acids work in your body at night.

Get more out of life with amino acids!

CHAPTER 7

Sleep

One of the most powerful healing processes that restore your health and wellbeing is sleep. When you sleep, your body goes through the process of resetting itself and replacing worn out tissue with new healthy tissue. By breaking down old tissue during sleep, free-form amino acids are released from your muscle, bone and liver into the blood stream, and used for the rebuilding and healing process. Supplementation can augment their levels and increase the benefits.

The roles of amino acids during sleep include:

- Rebuilding and renewing cells throughout the body.

- Storing up a good reserve of amino acids for the brain's neurotransmitters that maintain our mood, sleep and focus.
- Supporting processes that remove chemical toxins that may have accumulated during the day.
- Supporting the natural sleep state so that all those other processes can go on.

Among the amino acids essential for good sleep is tryptophan. Among its many functions, tryptophan is an essential precursor to the neurotransmitter serotonin, which in turn is the precursor to melatonin, and melatonin is a neural regulator that promotes deep, prolonged sleep. As evening falls and light gets dim, the body has an innate mechanism that transforms serotonin into melatonin and initiates sleep. Many users of tryptophan supplements find that this alone is a good sleep aid, but it does not substitute for the functions of all the other amino acids.

A complete blend must have tryptophan in it as one of the 22 amino acids. Some broad spectrum formulas have only 15 to 18 amino acids in them. I have found these to be good for some athletic performance programs, but not for brain and central nervous system health. In fact, taking amino acid formulas that lack tryptophan for long periods has apparently been known to lead to depression for some individuals.

For best results, take the complete blend in the mid-afternoon and before bedtime. By taking a complete blend in the mid-afternoon, you are beginning to build the serotonin pool of neurotransmitters in your brain. Then, as the sun sets, you have a robust supply of the chemical that transforms into melatonin. The quality of sleep you get will be the determining factor whether this dose will be enough for you. If you should wake up during the night, the protocol has not necessarily failed, just keep some capsules at your bedside and take 2,350 mg more. Most reports I receive are that within 20 minutes you will find yourself fast asleep and back in the state of mind we need to be in for healing.

Other amino acids assisting you while you are sleeping are GABA for calming the brain, threonine for bringing the brain waves into a theta wavelength, and taurine, which regulates and controls the nerve impulses throughout the nervous system. The amino acid glycine is a brain enhancer, arginine aids in wound healing and in building human growth hormone, and tyrosine is required in building thyroid hormone. The thyroid gland is the body's chief metabolic regulator. It is well known that if your thyroid is out of balance it can lead to sluggish metabolism and depression and/or sleep disorders can follow.

Disrupted sleep patterns, too little, too much, or at the wrong times of day, are common. If you suffer any of these symptoms your attention and performance are likely to be impaired in addition to the discomfort you feel, so try some of these strategies:

- *Restore a healthy association between your bed and sleep.* Establish the bed and bedroom as dedicated to rest. Don't introduce other activities like reading, writing, television, etc., into your mind's association with the bed. When you go to bed, let the mind automatically trigger the sleep cycle. If you don't fall asleep within 20-30 minutes of going to bed try getting up and doing some quiet activity elsewhere rather than allowing the bed to become associated with restlessness and frustration.

- *Use light and dark effectively.* In the day, use light to trigger wakefulness. In the evening use dark to trigger sleep. If your brain is fully activated during the day it will be easier to fall asleep at night, and a modest amount of sunlight early in the day is very helpful setting the biological clock. Avoid bright lights in the evening so that the night half of the cycle is not interrupted.

- *Hide the clock.* If you awaken during the night don't bother with the time, you already know that it's time for sleep. Focusing on the clock would only bring you to more alertness, the opposite of what you need. If you notice that you're focusing on anything at all, just let it go and be assured that it doesn't need to be analyzed in bed. Relax; with quality sleep you will be able to do a better job with it in the morning.

- *Use free-form amino acids effectively.* A complete blend is best for supporting overall brain health including the sleep function. If needed, a little extra tryptophan can be taken to enhance both mood and sleep. Small amounts (0.5 to 3 mg) of supplemental melatonin can help initiate sleep, but if the other amino acids are inadequately supplied, the effect may wear off and sleep interruption can occur a few hours later. For some people excessively large doses of melatonin can have an activating rather than calming effect, so you must find the correct dose for your specific metabolic needs.

- *If you wake up, don't worry.* As mentioned earlier, it is okay to take a little more of a complete blend and go back to bed. Try not to worry about insomnia, just relax and think, "Aaah… sweet rest."

When you master deep, prolonged sleep, the problems discussed in the next chapter regarding emotional eating and carbohydrate cravings will become ever so much easier to overcome!

***Remember—amino acids are foundation builders.
A good night's sleep starts there!***

CHAPTER 8

Emotional Eating, Carbohydrate Craving

In my 25-year practice, I have observed a great many patients, as well as others in the general public, who struggle with emotional eating. While uncovering the layers of amino acid benefits, I discovered their potential to also address emotional eating issues. Emotional eating is the practice of consuming large quantities of food, usually comfort or junk foods, in response to their feelings instead of hunger. One registered dietician has expressed an opinion that 75% of overeating is caused by emotions. [56]

Many of us learn that food can bring comfort, at least in the short term. As a result, we often turn to food to suppress emotional problems. Eating becomes a habit preventing us from learning skills and taking action that can effectively resolve our emotional distress. Depression, boredom, loneliness, anxiety, chronic anger, stress, frustration, problems with interpersonal relationships, and poor self-esteem can result in overeating and unwanted weight gain.

By identifying what triggers our eating, we can substitute more appropriate techniques to manage our emotional problems and take food and weight gain out of the equation. By learning how amino acids and other micronutrients can aid to heal, detoxify and balance your brain's chemistry, you will find your efforts bring quicker, more lasting results.

How can I identify eating triggers?

Situations and emotions that trigger us to eat fall into five main categories:

- *Social.* Eating when around other people. For example: excessive eating can result from being encouraged by others to eat, eating to fit in, arguing, or feelings of inadequacy around other people.
- *Emotional.* Eating in response to boredom, stress, fatigue, tension, depression, anger, anxiety or loneliness as a way to "fill the void."
- *Situational.* Eating because the opportunity is there. For example: at a restaurant, seeing an advertisement for a particular food or passing by a bakery and craving what you see. Eating may also be associated with certain activities such as watching TV, going to the movies or a sporting event, etc.
- *Thoughts.* Eating as a result of negative self-worth or making excuses for eating. For example: scolding oneself for looks or a lack of will power.

- *Physiological.* Eating in response to physical cues. For example: increased hunger due to skipping meals or eating to cure headaches or other pain.

I find the following narrative interesting and helpful in that it relates a holistic practitioner's professional experience in helping her patients work through and overcome these problems.

THE CORRECTIVE EXPERIENCE
By Judy Chang, Ph.D.

As a holistic psychologist who specializes in reducing emotional cravings, chemical addictions and substance abuse, I have a multi-factorial approach to working with my clients. A few of the most common and universal recommendations are life style changes such as regular pleasurable physical activity, nutrition and supplements. This normally includes a wide spectrum of vitamin and mineral micronutrients containing plenty of antioxidants, B vitamins, and other essential nutrients to support proper brain function. It will also often include a wide spectrum amino acid supplementation. Everyone is recommended Omega 3 fatty acids in the form of fish oil and probiotics, either through food or supplements.

I also address any addictions and use of mood-altering substances, including the use of any prescribed psychotropic medication that the client might be using. I look for possible toxins the client may be taking into his or her system and try to address that. I will use the client's sense of spirituality as a resource in our work together. I also consider the effects of EMR (electro-magnetic radiation) on our subtle bio-energy system and recommend ways of protecting ourselves from them.

In terms of my therapeutic approach, in addition to more traditional psychotherapy, I use a great deal of EMDR (Eye Movement Desensitization and Reprocessing). I also add something I call Alchemy to my work which is a transformational process. The work is focused on transforming negative experiences, memories, feelings and beliefs into positive ones. I like to think of my approach as being similar to being a transplant surgeon, removing the bad organ and replacing it with a good one. I think it's important in most cases to have the corrective experience.

So much of traditional psychiatric medicine treats the symptoms without addressing the cause, whether that cause is from some traumatic event(s) or improper or inadequate nutrition. Most emotional eaters, addicts and alcoholics are attempting to self-medicate. In either case, medication without addressing the cause of the distress is like buying a pair of jeans on your credit card and never paying it off. The debt becomes bigger and bigger until it becomes unmanageable. Sooner or later, you have to face the debt and deal with it.

Focusing on having the corrective experience helps to make something that is scary and overwhelming manageable, and yes, even, pleasurable. Some of the deepest tears are those of joy, because they get to experience, for the first time, what it was they had always needed.

Overcoming Carbohydrate Cravings

If you find that no matter how much you try to overcome carbohydrate cravings or emotional eating and are still unsuccessful, realize you are not the only one. Food has a quality to sooth our mood, comfort our feelings and make us feel like we are not deprived.

However, there are better options than excess food for controlling those feelings. Research demonstrates that many addictive behaviors or patterns can successfully be treated with the amino acids found in a complete blend. Specifically, tryptophan, glutamine, phenylalanine, and GABA have a robust impact on curbing many addictive behaviors.

I observed routinely in private practice with my patients who have had emotional eating tendencies that, while taking a complete blend, they experienced:

- Fewer cravings for carbohydrates
- A reduced incidence of stress
- An increased likelihood of recovery, and
- Reduction in relapse rates

The key to overcoming emotional eating is to restore and regulate normal neurotransmitter balance. In this section we will look at the most common substances used when we are emotionally eating, sugar, fat, salt, caffeine, nicotine, and alcohol, and how to break free of them.

The good news is that there's a healthy fix that works in restoring your maximum brain function with no withdrawal or other negative side effects. Since the brain's communication system works with chemicals that are made from nutrients, amino acids, vitamins, and minerals, we can formulate the perfect "brain food" to restore them, and break the cycle of addiction. Nutritional supplements can be used to aid in healing your brain and create a state of high energy as well as increased focus.

You will recover much faster from substance reliance if you use specific supplements to restore your brain's chemical balance. Why? There are millions of chemical reactions that occur every second in every cell of your body. These very important reactions require specific nutrients in order to function properly. Particularly sensitive are our neurons or nerve cells, which require just the right raw materials to manufacture our neurotransmitters (chemical messengers that control our mind, mood, and behavior). When we don't have the raw materials we need, we become depressed, drowsy, irritable, or agitated, or we can't think or concentrate properly.

The key to overcoming emotional eating is to supply your brain cells with the nutrients it needs that satiate the cravings for sugars, sweets, fats, nicotine, prescription medications and/or recreational drugs. In addition, I frequently also refer my patients to a certified EDMR therapist (Eye Movement Desensitization and Reprocessing). This style of therapy can rapidly aid to transform the patient's belief system so that they get back in charge. It allows a quick response to overcome long term self-doubt and low self-esteem. A combination of EDMR therapy and micronutrients supplementation is a powerful model for finding your path to success.

Detoxification

Once you have the mindset to make changes to overcome emotional eating, your next step is to follow "The Amino Detox" protocol. *See Appendix C: Amino Detoxification.*

Remember: amino acids fuel the cellular machinery to detoxify the toxic chemicals in your brain that led to the chronic tendency to overeat in the first place. Once these amino acids are saturated in the cells of your brain, the brain will begin to reset itself and cravings should be greatly reduced. The reason for this is once the DNA in the nucleus of the cell is fueled with the amino acids needed to reset itself, the DNA will stop sending messengers out for the toxic addictive chemicals it once thought were normal. The amino acids not only fuel the missing link of needed nutrients to the DNA, they also aid to detoxify the environment in the cell, which resulted from poor eating habits.

"The Amino Detox" protocol aids to decrease the carbohydrate cravings and to detoxify the chemical waste that is stored in the cells. This is why I saw such dramatic results in my private practice when utilizing amino acids with patients suffering from emotional eating.

If you've had a history of any autoimmune disorders, such as liver, kidney, spleen, or heart disease you should discuss the integration of any detox program with your healthcare professional prior to beginning.

Amino acids are naturally powerful detoxifiers!

CHAPTER 9

Substance Abuse
and Chemical Dependency

I have watched many people come into recovery and just as quickly, they disappear, only to come back again and again, claiming a desire to get better. What causes them to go through that revolving door for so long?

Addiction is a multifaceted issue typically involving harmful substances, but also emotional adversities and unhealthy lifestyles. Common illegal, harmful addictions include marijuana, cocaine, heroin, ecstasy and a myriad of other "recreational" drugs. But equally as devastating to one's health and well-being are addictions to other, legal substances, such as alcohol, prescription drugs such as antidepressants and pain killers, tobacco, caffeine, simple sugars, high glycemic index carbohydrates, chocolate, cocoa, and trans fatty acid foods. What is causing us to need or crave these substances? The answer begins in that fantastically complex sphere we call the brain. Not our actual thinking, but our brain chemistry itself.

When the neurotransmitters are depleted or are being reabsorbed by our brain's receptor sites too quickly, we reach automatically for something that will make us feel better. This can be achieved through many substances and is especially true of alcohol. It is a legal "fix" to our continuing feelings of restlessness, irritability and discontentment. Unfortunately any of these temporary fixes (alcohol, antidepressants, caffeine, simple sugars, artificial sweeteners, chocolate, cocoa, etc.) only mask the cause of the problem which remains unaddressed due to addictive chemical imbalance and behaviors.

Amino acid therapy has proven extraordinarily robust in its performance in recovery from substance abuse, chemical dependency and in medication reduction or what is called titration. There are multiple research studies demonstrating how and why the amino acid support works.

Research done by Kenneth Blum, Ph.D., at the University of North Texas, demonstrates that the brain chemistry of alcoholics and drug addicts includes a few genes that can cause the brain to under produce the neurotransmitters needed to stabilize individuals' moods. His research explains why feelings of anxiety, frustration, and depression plague so many addicts. Dr. Blum called this genetic deficit phenomenon the

"Reward Deficiency Syndrome." His research also showed that by providing his patients with amino acid therapy, they were significantly more capable of refraining from drug and alcohol use.

What is it that causes our brains to lose the ability to naturally take care of ourselves via neurotransmission? Research shows us the answer is deficiency, plain and simple. It can be a deficiency in any number of nutrients, trace elements or essential fatty acids, but primarily in the case of addiction, it is typically a deficiency in the amino acid tyrosine. Deficiencies of this amino acid can cause cravings for caffeine, speed, cocaine, marijuana, concentrated simple sugars, fructose, sucrose, sugars, aspartame (artificial sweetener), high fructose corn syrup, chocolate, cocoa, alcohol, tobacco, and starches. Symptoms of tyrosine deficiency are depression, low energy, lack of focus and concentration and attention deficit disorder.

If a person is suffering from any of those symptoms, they are naturally going to reach for substances that will allow them to feel better, even if only for a short time. This is why many individuals find themselves taking antidepressants. Unfortunately, antidepressants do little more than slow down the re-absorption of certain neurotransmitters. The individual might feel better, but it never takes care of the underlying problem, and can be harmful to our physical health if taken for long periods of time.

A study entitled "The Hypoascorbemia-Kwashiorkor Approach to Drug Addiction Therapy: A Pilot Study" (Alfred F. Libby and Irwin Stone; Australas NursJ. 1978 Jan-Feb; 7 (6) 4-8, 13. PMID: 4187640) demonstrates the essential need of taking amino acids, sodium ascorbate and a multi-vitamin/mineral to effectively manage chronic substance abuse.

A different solution, which actually addresses the underlying problem, is to receive adequate amounts of amino acids, sodium ascorbate and a high quality multi-vitamin mineral Into our bodies. This can be achieved through eating a healthy diet and supplementation.

To assist the recovery, I also highly recommend an amino detoxification (*see Appendix B: Amino Detoxification*) with the following additions:

- To assist in amino acid nutritional therapy, the use of sodium ascorbate and a multivitamin/mineral formula is recommended. Many vitamins and minerals serve as cofactors in neurotransmitter synthesis. They also serve to restore general balance, vitality and wellbeing to those who typically are in a state of poor nutritional health.

The chart immediately following provides additional information regarding symptoms of addiction with their specific amino acid deficiency.

Amino acids are important underlying components to sustainable recovery!

AMINO ACID NUTRITION THERAPY

Supplemental Ingredient	Restored Brain Chemical	Addictive Substance Abuse	Amino Acid Deficiency Symptoms	Expected Behavior Change
D-Phenylalanine or DL-Phenylalanine	Enkephalins Endorphins	Heroin, Alcohol, Marijuana, Sweets, Starches, Chocolate, Tobacco	Most Reward Deficiency Syndrome (RDS) conditions sensitive to physical or emotional pain. Crave comfort and pleasure. Desire certain food or drugs.	Anti-craving. Mild anti-depression. Mild improved energy & focus. Promotes pain relief, increases pleasure.
L-Phenylalanine or L-Tyrosine	Norepinephrine Dopamine	Caffeine, Speed, Cocaine, Marijuana, Aspartame, Chocolate, Alcohol, Tobacco, Starches	Most Reward Deficiency Syndrome (RDS) conditions. Depression, low energy. Lack of focus and concentration. Attention-deficit disorder.	Reward stimulation. Anti-depression. Increased energy. Improved focus.
L-Tryptophan or 5 hydroxytryptophan (5HTP)	Serotonin	Sweets, Alcohol, Starch, Ecstasy, Marijuana, Chocolate, Tobacco	Low self-esteem. Obsessive/compulsive behaviors. Irritability or rage. Sleep problems. Afternoon or evening cravings. Negativity. Heat intolerance. Fibromyalgia, SAD (winter blues).	Anti-craving. Anti-depression. Anti-insomnia. Improved appetite control. Improvement in mood & other serotonin deficiency symptoms.
GABA (Gamma-amino butyric acid)	GABA	Valium, Alcohol, Marijuana, Tobacco, Sweets, Starches	Feeling of being stressed-out. Nervous. Tense muscles. Trouble relaxing.	Promotes calmness. Promotes relaxation.
L-Glutamine	GABA (mild enhancement) Fuel source for entire brain	Sweets, Starches, Alcohol	Stress. Mood swings. Hypoglycemia.	Anti-craving, anti-stress. Levels blood sugar and mood. GABA (mild enhancement). Fuel source for entire brain.

Note: To assist in amino-acid nutritional therapy, the use of a multi-vitamin/mineral formula is recommended. Many vitamins and minerals serve as co-factors in neurotransmitter synthesis. They also serve to restore general balance, vitality and well-being to the Reward Deficiency Syndrome (RSD) patient who typically is in a state of poor nutritional health.

This chart was originally published in the following article.
Blum K, Ross J, Reuben C, Gastelu D, Miller DK. "Nutritional Gene Therapy: Natural Healing in Recovery. Counselor Magazine, January/February, 2001

This chart was originally published in: Blum K, Ross J, Reuben C, Gastelu D, Miller DK. "Nutritional Gene Therapy: Natural Healing in Recovery. Counselor Magazine, January/February, 2001.

CHAPTER 10

Chronic Emotional and Physical Pain, Wound Healing, Fibromyalgia

As a health care professional, I have found that one of the most challenging experiences with family, friends and patients is witnessing the chronic emotional and physical pain people go through at different times in their lives. So, when I began to see in my private practice the amazing results my patients were achieving with the use of a complete blend as a therapeutic modality, I had to dig deep in the research to learn why.

I'm going to share with you a few concepts to lay a foundation of understanding so that the simple answer can make more sense. The fact is we all know someone who is suffering from chronic physical or emotional pain. We naturally want to help them help themselves. Our body was designed to have a natural capacity to heal, but it must first obtain the essential nutrients required for healing from food and supplements. The opposite is true as well: when our bodies do not have all the nutrients required to heal, the healing process is slowed or halted.

In relation to amino acids, this concept can mean several things:

1. A hidden amino acid deficiency can lead to multiple physical and emotional difficulties plus a variety of other symptoms.
2. A complete blend can easily and safely alleviate hidden amino acid deficiencies.
3. Symptoms of amino acid deficiencies are rapidly reduced or cleared utilizing a complete blend.

Having an understanding that the body can heal itself when the right nutrients are available, we can then appreciate the importance of supplying all the amino acids required to build certain chemicals the body needs to heal. In regards to the chronic emotional and physical pain many of us deal with, we need to look to the body's natural pain reducing chemicals called endorphins. Endorphins require over 15 amino acids as a precursor to synthesize them [56]. This is the beauty behind a complete blend; it has all 22 amino acids in a well-balanced formula.

Endorphins are our body's natural morphine. When someone is very ill or has had a serious injury or surgery, doctors will often prescribe morphine as a saving grace to relieve acute pain. Morphine is a poor long term solution because it creates many other problems. The body naturally makes endorphins to manage pain and morphine only simulates them.

However, in life, we may have to deal with long term emotional and or physical pain for a variety of reasons. Initially, when you have an injury or an emotional trauma, your body will supply you with plenty of endorphins to assist in reducing the degree of pain you experience. The problem is, if the pain continues week after week, month after month, and year after year, your body uses up the endorphin supplies. *It is very difficult to get enough amino acids in your daily dietary intake to maintain the level of endorphins needed to deal with chronic emotional and or physical pain.*

The beauty of a complete blend is that you can take a daily supply. This fuels your body with ample amino acids needed to increase your endorphins, the body's natural morphine supply.

Is this the cure all? In some cases, yes. Is it for all illnesses and pain conditions? Unfortunately, it is not. However, I am very impressed with the ability of these amino acids to reduce chronic emotional and physical pain. Because results can be so individualized, I recommend a person trying a therapeutic dosage of a complete blend *(see Appendix A: How to Take Amino Acids)* for a six week period to learn what degree of chronic pain is actually reduced.

Additionally you will want to take:

- A high-quality, chelated mineral supplement at breakfast and lunch
- 400 to 800 mg of omega 3 fish oils
- A high-quality probiotic
- A high grade, loose green tea, four to six times per day

If after two weeks into the program you are not feeling a reduction in pain, you will want to add to your supplement intake 500 to 1000 mg of the individual amino acid, dl-phenylalanine (DLPA). DLPA works as a booster to endorphin levels because d-phenylalanine apparently suppresses the rate of endorphin breakdown.

Note: If you experience chronic pain you may also want to be checked out to see whether you are gluten intolerant. If you should discover that you are gluten intolerant, you may be one of the many who can benefit from a gluten-free diet. A combination of a gluten-free diet and the amino acid supplement protocol mentioned above is a smart choice.

Back Pain and More

Many health care professionals recommend a therapeutic dosage for physical conditions such as chronic back, neck and shoulder pain, TMJ syndrome, headaches, arthritic pain and stiffness, wound healing and more. This dosage is also used by health care professionals to alleviate mood disorders, anxiety, etc.

Wound Healing

The immune system also plays a role in the early stages of wound healing. It is responsible for preparing damaged tissue for repair and promoting the recruitment of certain cells to the wound area. Consistent with the fact that stress alters the production of cytokines, it has been discovered that chronic stress associated with care giving for a person with Alzheimer's disease leads to delayed wound healing. Research results indicate that biopsy wounds healed 25% more slowly in the chronically stressed group and those caring for a person with Alzheimer's disease, than in the unstressed control group.

Other risk factors for delayed wound healing include:

- Arthritis
- Chronic liver disease
- Diabetes
- Excess alcohol intake
- Impaired self-caring
- Inadequate nutrition
- Inflammatory disease
- Older age (over 65 years)
- Poor circulation
- Poor cognition/cognitive dysfunction
- Renal failure
- Smoking
- Vascular disease
- Weakened immune system[218]

Opposing these risk factors, amino acids and other micronutrients are well documented for aiding in wound healing. How? Wound healing requires the body to replace injured tissue with new tissue, which requires increased consumption of nutrients, particularly protein and calories. Improved nutritional status enables the body to heal wounds faster,[61] and accelerated wound healing has actually been observed with nutritional supplementation. [62-63] As you have already learned, amino acids are the building blocks of protein; you cannot rebuild tissue without them. These are some of ways free-form amino acids aiding in wound healing:

1. Nutrition profoundly influences the process of wound healing. Nutritional depletion exerts an inhibitory effect, and nutritional supplementation with such positive effectors as arginine can stimulate wound healing. [64]

2. The use of glutamine and arginine supplements enhances woundhealingandshouldbeincreased.Nutritionalcareiscost-effective. (65)

3. "Arginine ... is involved with protein synthesis ... with cell signalling through the production of nitric oxide and cell proliferation through its metabolism to ornithine and the other polyamines. Because of these multiple functions, arginine is an essential substrate for wound healing processes. The requirement for this amino acid in tissue repair is highlighted." (66)

With amino acids, I have personally seen many successful outcomes in several different types of wounds that would otherwise not heal. If you have a stubborn lesion, a burn or an ulcer, you may want to take free-form amino acid supplements for four to six weeks and observe if this helps to speed the wound healing process. I recommend that you take 2,350 mg complete blend amino acid, four times per day, for four to six weeks to see if this improves the wound. Always discuss any changes in your recovery process/approach with your health care professional.

Wound healing via amino acid support is a relatively new modality and is just one more of the latest researched areas affected by stress that benefit from broad spectrum, free-form amino acid supplementation.

Understanding Fibromyalgia

Fibromyalgia is a disease of widespread soft tissue pain and stiffness. It often coincides with symptoms of persistent fatigue, exercise intolerance, disrupted sleep, tension headaches, migraines, blurred vision, abnormalities of the skin or fingernails, painful menstrual periods, numbness or tingling, heart palpitations, sleep apnea, temperature sensitivity, restless legs, impaired cognition, irritable bladder, and irritable intestinal symptoms.

Fibromyalgia affects an estimated six million Americans and accounts for $9 billion annually in conventional medical care and another $13 billion in alternative treatments like naturopathy, acupuncture and massage therapy. Sixty percent of cases are diagnosed between ages 30 and 50, eighty to ninety percent of which are in women. (57-58)·

Fibromyalgia is characterized by chronic widespread pain and tenderness for at least 3 months. Currently there are no diagnostic tests, such as x-rays or blood tests, to detect fibromyalgia. The symptoms of fibromyalgia may overlap with the symptoms of other conditions. That is why fibromyalgia is sometimes difficult to diagnose.

Some healthcare providers use guidelines set by the American College of Rheumatology to help make a diagnosis.

These guidelines include if a person has had both:

- Chronic widespread pain that affects the right and left sides of the body above and below the waist.
- Pain in at least 11 of 18 possible tender points, (nine on one side of the body, nine on the other), when light pressure is applied.

Your healthcare provider may use these guidelines or other methods to make a diagnosis of fibromyalgia. Discuss all of your symptoms with your healthcare provider. Talk openly with him or her about what you are feeling and how your symptoms are affecting you. You can work together to create a plan that meets your individual needs and helps you manage your symptoms.

Fibromyalgia may be related to protein and essential nutrient deficiencies. [59] If the availability of amino acids and other essential micronutrients is insufficient to adequately maintain or repair muscle tissue, then collagen may be the body's best alternative for providing structural support in spite of a loss of normal muscle structure/function. The stiffness and pain associated with fibromyalgia may be the result of structural abnormalities resulting from the replacement of one tissue type with another.

It's not surprising that soft tissue degeneration and ill health result when protein ingestion, digestion or assimilation is deficient. This is especially true when there is an ongoing deficiency of quality food intake, thus lacking the essential nutrients the body needs for healing and repair.

If you decide to try broad spectrum amino acid supplementation for fibromyalgia, it is essential to combine high quality vitamin, mineral, vitamin C, omega 3 fatty acids and probiotic supplements into your plan. The amino acids require all the essential nutrients from other supplements to heal and repair the skeletal muscle damage, strengthen your immune system and balance the brains neurotransmitters to optimize the recovery process. This regimen may need to be followed for six to twelve months.

When it comes to chronic physical and emotional pain, amino acids are the fuel for your body's endorphin needs!

CHAPTER 11

Stress and Post Traumatic Stress Disorder (PTSD)

Stress

It is always a challenge to help patients recover from their primary complaints of sleeplessness, anxiety, depression, back pain or muscle fatigue when their stress level is elevated. I have found the most stressed patients are single mothers, patients who have just broken up with a loved one, have had a recent death in the family, or loss of a career. This level of pressure put on anyone is enough to cause such tension that most therapies, at best, yield temporary relief.

When I started recommending to my patients that they begin to take 2,350 mg of a complete amino acid blend, two to four times a day, I began to see real leveling of the underlying symptoms and distress. How exactly do amino acids accomplish this?

Let's look at how the body works with stress. As you have learned from previous chapters, the amino acids are the building blocks for all the neurotransmitters in the brain and central nervous system. Research indicates that medium to high levels of stress can result in up to a 60% increase in burning all available micronutrients in your body within a 24-hour period [(60)]. It makes sense that you will need to restore these micronutrients (amino acids, vitamins, and minerals) to assure your body is being taken care of as result of the depletion. Because stress can lower your immune strength, it also makes sense to double up on your supplements during stressful times.

Homeostasis, maintenance of a steady state, is a concept central to the idea of stress. In biology, most biochemical processes strive to maintain equilibrium, a steady state that exists more as an ideal and less as an achievable condition. Environmental factors, internal or external stimuli, continually push the system away from this steady state. Thus, an organism's condition is in a state of constant flux wavering about a homeostatic point that would be that organism's optimal condition for living.

Factors causing this condition to waver away from homeostasis can be interpreted as stress. In such instances, an organism's fight or flight response recruits the body's energy stores and focuses its attention to overcome the challenge at hand.

Because stress has so many subjective factors, its definition is subjective as well. First to use the term in a biological context, Hans Selye defined stress as, "the non-specific response of the body to any demand placed upon it." Present day neuroscientist Jaap Koolhass believes, based on years of empirical research, that the term stress, "should be restricted to conditions where an environmental demand exceeds the natural regulatory capacity of an organism." What does that mean exactly? That sometimes our circumstances push us beyond our capacity to cope and we suffer the symptoms of stress. In relation to how amino acids assist in leveling the symptoms of stress, we can consider the many different systems in our body that stress affects. *See Appendix D: Figure 4.2.*

The Brain, Spinal Cord, and Stress

The brain plays a critical role in the body's perception of and response to stress. Pinpointing exactly which regions of the brain are responsible for particular aspects of a stress response is difficult and often unclear. Understanding that the brain works in more of a network-like fashion carrying information about a stressful situation across regions of the brain, from cortical sensory areas to more basal structures and vice-versa, can help explain how stress and its negative consequences are heavily rooted in dysfunctions of neural communication.

The spinal cord, then, plays the critical role of transferring stress response neural impulses from the brain to the rest of the body. The spinal cord communicates with the rest of the body by connecting the brain to the peripheral nervous system. Certain nerves that belong to the sympathetic branch of the central nervous system exit the spinal cord and stimulate peripheral nerves, which in turn engage the body's major organs and muscles in a fight or flight manner. In addition, the neuroendocrine blood hormone signaling system initiated by the hypothalamus sends out stimulating chemical messengers.

When a person experiences stress, neurotransmitters are signaled. These neurotransmitters relay positive and negative message responses to the brain *through the spinal cord*. When released, endorphins, (a class of neurotransmitters made up of amino acids) naturally regulate signals indicating pain or stress. This is your body's natural defense to stress, and it requires a healthy spinal cord and amino acids to function properly.

Remember, the amino acids are the building blocks for all the chemicals for communications and signaling in the brain and nervous system. When you include them in your wellbeing regime, you are in fact offering first aid to improve the nutrients that fortify the chemicals that assure all your body's communication lines are fueled.

The Effect of Stress on the Immune System

Research has shown that stress has a definite, negative effect on the immune system. Most of that was through studies in which participants were subjected to certain viruses. In one study, individuals caring for a spouse with dementia, representing the stress group, saw a significant decrease in immune response when given an influenza virus vaccine, compared to a non-stressed control group. Another study was conducted using a respiratory virus. Participants were infected with the virus and given a stress index. Results showed that an increase in score on the stress index correlated with greater severity of cold symptoms. Studies with HIV have also shown that stress tends to speed up viral progression. Men with HIV were two to three times more likely to progress into full blown AIDS when they were under above average stress.

When a complete blend enters the bloodstream, the first priority it attends to is to check in and see if your immune system is under undue stress. If it is, the essential and non-essential amino acids go to work to give your immune system all the support it needs. As a matter of survival, your body's natural intelligence wants to stop any type of infectious disease before it can establish a stronghold in your system. Therefore the body will prioritize the immune system when free-form amino acids become available. Many of my clients take a complete blend as a wellness and prevention product just for this reason.

Chronic Stress

Chronic stress is defined as a "state of prolonged tension from internal or external stressors, which may cause various physical manifestations, for example: asthma, back pain, arrhythmias, fatigue, headaches, irritable bowel syndrome and ulcers, and suppress the immune system."

Chronic stress takes a more significant toll on your body than acute stress does. It can raise blood pressure, increase the risk of heart attack and stroke, increase vulnerability to anxiety and depression, contribute to infertility, and hasten the aging process.

Results of one study demonstrated that individuals who reported relationship conflict lasting one month or longer have a greater risk of developing illness and show slower wound healing. Similarly, the effects that acute stressors have on the immune system may be increased when there is perceived stress and/or anxiety due to other events. For example, students who are taking exams show weaker immune responses if they also report feeling stress due to daily hassles.

In most cases, what we see with chronic stress is chronic emotional and/or physical pain. In chronic stress conditions the stress will ultimately use up the endorphins. You will need to rebuild your endorphin supply, which is made up of amino acids. The endorphins are your body's natural morphine. By taking a complete blend you are assisting to refuel your depleted endorphins, as well as your overall immune health.

Post-Traumatic Stress Disorder (PTSD)

As I mentioned earlier in the chapter on anxiety, prior to amino acid therapy, I often experienced deep, unresolved anxiousness in certain settings of my life. Although therapy was essential and allowed me to let parts of myself feel free, whole, and independent in my adult life, I still had not been able to integrate that sense of wholeness constantly. I am not talking about the anxiety due to routine living; I am talking about an anxiousness that carries over from the past, which would frequently plague me and impair my experience of daily living. Through the years I came to understand that I was dealing with a form of post-traumatic stress disorder (PTSD).

As I learned about and began taking the amino acids and other essential nutrients that balance the brain and nervous system, I was finally able to integrate all the great insights that I developed from the challenging work of therapy. All my efforts to heal that resulted in a successful integration of psychotherapeutic experience with essential nutrient supplementation led to results so powerful that I developed a deep passion to pass this knowledge on to my patients and other healthcare professionals. My experience is somewhat unusual. I did not learn about amino acids and their powerful effect from textbook reading. I had firsthand experience and recovery. After applying this knowledge to my patient's care, with amazing and constant results, I naturally began lecturing on the broad topic I call, "Micronutrients for Physical and Mental Health," which has inspired even more research into the effects of amino acid supplementation on PTSD.

It is estimated that the classical diagnostic criteria for PTSD occurs in about 3.6% of adult Americans—about 5.2 million people during the course of a year. If we were able to count the number of people worldwide who experienced PTSD at some point in their lives, the number would be staggering. It is estimated that 10 to 30% of war veterans will suffer from some form of PTSD. Women are more than 2.5 times as likely as men to develop PTSD.

PTSD usually occurs within three months of the event, but in some it might not occur until years later. Severity and duration of the disabling symptoms vary and recovery may take months or years depending on the recognition and proper treatment of the disorder. Shock, anger, nervousness, fear, guilt and other similar symptoms are common after any traumatic event. What distinguishes the PTSD sufferer is that they become disabled by these symptoms and have them with greater severity and duration than most of us.

Treatment can include lifestyle modifications, nutrition, reduction in psychosocial stresses, individual or group psychotherapies that address current, past developmental and trauma issues, and interventions as suggested by lab testing. Lab testing may lead to the treatment of vitamin, mineral, amino acid, essential fatty acid or hormone deficiencies. Problems with digestive function or of pathologic organisms in the gut, or environmental issues as allergies and food sensitivities, or toxic metal problems may also be included in treatment.

The value of taking a complete blend for all degrees of stress on the body is four-fold:

1. By fuelling the body with the essential and non-essential amino acids in a balanced formula that is easily digestible, you offer a foundation to energize all the body's metabolic pathways that may become depleted from long-term stress.
2. In a stressful environment, the body will "steal from Peter to give to Paul." Supplying broad spectrum amino acids relieves the body of this imbalance.

3. PTSD and anxiety lead to gastrointestinal issues, which further impair the absorption of nutrients from our food. Amino acids are the precursor to digestive enzymes made in the pancreas; thus, when they are depleted, the enzymes can't be made and even further absorption problems result. Free-form amino acids can greatly help reduce this repetitive cycle.

4. Vitamins and minerals, which are essential in all cells of the body for effective amino acid transformation, are used up more rapidly under stress. Under these conditions some non-essential amino acids (contained in a compete blend) become conditionally essential.

Along with a well-balanced diet and drinking ample amounts of water, proper nutrient supplementation aid in resisting the intensive stress on the body and brain that result from PTSD. For maximum results take 2,350 mg of complete amino blend, four times per day, along with a high quality chelated vitamin/mineral, omega 3 fish oil and a probiotic at breakfast and lunch. You may need to add additional branched chain amino acid supplementation for moderate and severe PTSD. Branched chain amino acids specifically have had successful outcomes in recent research for PTSD and Traumatic Brain Injury. [67]

The amazing amino acids have far reaching benefits that are still being uncovered, system by system!

CHAPTER 12

New Frontiers for the Amazing Amino Acids: Mental Health, Medication Withdrawal, Diabetes, Optimal Health

Research is constantly emerging in new frontiers to support the paramount importance of integrating amino acids into our wellness and prevention approaches. New opportunities for amino acid therapy are being revealed as quickly as the science can unveil their healing attributes.

Mental Health

In September 2011 I had the honor of being a guest speaker at the Micronutrients for Mental Health Conference held at the New

York Academy of Medicine in Manhattan, New York. I was privileged to mingle with professionals and researchers, all leading experts in the field of integrative and mental health from around the world. The prevalent topic: integration of the entire micronutrient family as a nutritional therapy for mental health. I was greatly intrigued. Remember, the micronutrient family includes:

- Amino acids
- Vitamins/Minerals
- Essential fatty acids

It is typical to find micronutrient deficiencies in patients with mood disorders, sleeplessness, autism, ADHD, and more. These emerging fields: "Integrative Psychiatry" and "Integrative Health Care," now offer patients an alternative to traditional prescription medication by recommending a combination of amino acids, vitamins, minerals, and essential fatty acids as a first line of defense.

One of the most common mental health conditions, ADHD, has shown promising results in clinical trials with the application of micronutrient therapy. According to a study performed by the Department of Psychology at the University of Canterbury, "Results suggest that micronutrients may increase resilience to ongoing stress and anxiety associated with a highly stressful event in individuals with ADHD and are consistent with controlled studies showing benefit of micronutrients for mental health." [68]

World-renown chemist and Nobel Peace Prize winner, Linus Pauling, explored the relationship of critical micronutrients and enzymes with mental illness. [69] Pauling proposed that mental abnormalities might be successfully treated by correcting imbalances or deficiencies among naturally occurring biochemical constituents of the brain, notably vitamins, and other micronutrients, including amino acids, as an alternative to the administration of potent, synthetic psychoactive drugs. [70]

Recent studies demonstrate that the branch chain amino acids (BCAA) reduce manic symptoms. [214] According to the Diagnostic and Statistical Manual of Mental Disorders, "a lack of certain dietary nutrients contribute to the development of mental disorders. Notably, essential vitamins, minerals, and omega 3 fatty acids are often deficient in the general population, and are exceptionally deficient in patients suffering from mental disorders." The manual surmises "Supplements that contain amino acids reduce symptoms, because they are converted to neurotransmitters that alleviate depression and other mental disorders. Based on emerging scientific evidence, this form of nutritional supplement treatment may be appropriate for controlling major depression, bipolar disorder, schizophrenia and anxiety disorders, eating disorders, attention deficit disorder/attention deficit hyperactivity disorder (ADD/ADHD), addiction, and autism."

Of course moderate-to-acute mood disorders and long-standing mental illnesses may require a combination of psychotropic medications and micronutrients to stabilize the condition. Current research suggests that there is incredible potential for an improvement in a variety of behavioral problems via micronutrient supplementation. "This alternative and effective therapeutic approach may eventually reduce or even eliminate the need for most psychiatric medications used today worldwide." [71] Although this is a promising approach to alleviating mental health symptoms, consult your personal physician or an integrative healthcare professional before introducing any significant changes to your diet, lifestyle, or medication use.

Medication Withdrawal

An additional benefit has presented itself in the course of amino acid research: the reduction of medication withdrawal symptoms. For many patients, withdrawal symptoms from psychotropic medications can feel just like the illness or worse. Thanks to integrative science, there are now promising options for these painful symptoms. "The amino acids that have been used at medicinal dosages for the purpose of restoring the patient back to a state of balance and give the patient a fighting chance during medication withdrawal are specialized in their actions." [79] *See page 66: Amino Acid Nutrition Therapy Chart.*

Some amino acids calm, some detoxify, and some excite. Which to pick, and how much to take depends on the medication being withdrawn. Without these amino acids to rebuild deficient neurotransmitters, people who have been taking psychotropic medications for years can have great difficulty during withdrawal with the symptoms that these medications are supposed to treat." [72]

A complete blend is the optimum choice for rebuilding these neurotransmitter deficiencies during withdrawal. Some observed advantages of using a complete blend to reduce symptoms from medication withdrawal include:

- alleviating prior deficiencies that necessitated drug interventions
- providing substrate for synthesis of calming neurotransmitters: GABA, glycine, tryptophan, threonine, taurine
- facilitating polypeptide neural messenger synthesis, satisfying multi-component receptors
- amino acids function as "detoxifiers"

In respect to mood disorders, substance abuse and chemical dependencies, many individuals find a combination of single, high dose, free-form amino acid supplement therapy combined with a complete blend is the best combination for their recovery and healing. (See your personal healthcare provider for help).

Diabetes

According to the 2011 National Diabetes Information Clearinghouse:

- 25.8 million children and adults in the U.S. have diabetes. That is 8.3% of the population.
- 18.8 million are diagnosed.
- 7.0 million are undiagnosed.
- In 2005–2008, based on fasting glucose or hemoglobin A1C (HbA1C) levels, 35% of U.S. adults ages 20 years or older are pre-diabetic as well as 50% of adults ages 65 years or older (an estimated 79 million American adults with prediabetes).
- Diabetes is the seventh leading cause of death listed on U.S. death certificates.

As much as we observe free-form amino acids are balancing neurotransmitters in your brain, fueling all the cells in your body, and optimizing your health, they are also directly assisting in the physiological balance of controlling your blood sugar. This has a direct impact on your mood, energy, focus and all around health.

As I've already discussed, the amino acids are the building blocks for all the cells, regulating all the systems in your body. Whereas the amino acid precursor for the neurotransmitter serotonin is tryptophan, there are 17 amino acids required for the synthesis of insulin. By fueling your body with a complete blend, you are supplying all the building blocks to generate this essential hormone.

In a study completed in 2003 at the Nutrition and Toxicology Research Institute Maastricht in the Netherlands, scientists observed, "the insulin response in long-term Type 2 diabetic patients following carbohydrate intake can be nearly tripled by co-ingestion of a free form amino acid/protein mixture." The study indicates that amino acid ingestion strongly enhances insulin secretion in diabetics.

Research on the benefits of eating healthy meals to stabilize your blood sugar is well documented. However, it is my contention that as amino acids and other essential micronutrients are researched we will find that protocols to aid in Type 2 diabetic individuals will benefit their all around health, reduction of the common symptoms of diabetes and hypoglycemia, and an improved stabilization of insulin secretion. Although there is a lot of new research needed to back this premise, it is, nevertheless, possible and even foreseeable.

Optimal Health

Bruce Ames, Ph.D., found 40 essential micronutrients that are key to good health. He also observed that even with just one micronutrient deficiency, the body's metabolic pathways would begin to become imbalanced and an onset of some degree of illness would begin.

What does this mean in regards to amino acid supplementation? Amino acids are extraordinary, and often overlooked nutrients that can many times be an effective stand alone therapy for many symptoms. However, Dr. Ames' research indicates that they can also be extraordinarily effective toward optimum health when taken in conjunction with the rest of the micronutrient family, including vitamins, minerals, and the essential fatty acids (omega 3). This concept of a micronutrient wellness trinity—the essential and nonessential amino acids, vitamins/minerals, and fatty acids—brings all the puzzle pieces together for optimal health.

Our bodies are composed of elements, water, amino acids, fatty acids, vitamins, minerals, and cofactors. All the parts of "us", enzymes, peptides, hormones, neurotransmitters, cells of all types, are built daily, from these essential elements. Without each one of these essentials the process of birth, growth, regeneration and repair falters or fails.

Other researchers working with vitamins, amino acids, and fatty acids have come to similar conclusions. There is no one element more essential than the whole. We are about our pieces and parts, and how these elements work together. When six elements are needed but only five are present, the cell or enzyme or hormone will not be made, or may be made in inadequate numbers, or with errors. In addition, excessive amounts of any single nutrient can imbalance body processes creating relative (too much/not enough) insufficiency of co-nutrients in a particular action/function. [73-76]

Each day our bodies must repair or replace aging and injured cells. When those essential elements are not present in the diet or are not present in sufficient amounts, the processes of replacement/repair malfunction result in degenerative disease or in some cases defective repair with damage to DNA. [77] The key to nutrient sufficiency and health is balanced amounts, enough, but not too much, of *all* elements needed for body structure and function.

Biochemical individuality also plays a role in how healthy we are or can be. In persons with impaired genetics, micronutrient supplementation may be of great benefit. Currently some 50 genetic diseases or predispositions to diseases, caused by defective enzymes, can be remedied by oral administration of one or more of the vitamins or minerals used as cofactors in the defective enzymes. [78]

Pregnancy, nursing, puberty, menopause, aging, tissue damage from accident or surgery, environmental assault (chemicals, toxins, even too much sunlight), poor diet, insufficient intake of protein, fresh fruits and vegetables, infectious diseases both acute and chronic, all increase our need for every essential nutrient, every day. Not only do we need to make sure our intake meets our need, our needs may actually change from day to day and year to year, from birth through old age. We must adapt our trinity intake as we adapt to aging, each micronutrient as essential as the others.

In my own practice, I take the trinity a step further, adding a high-quality probiotic, to ensure that gastrointestinal issues do not hinder the benefits or impact of taking the full spectrum of micronutrients. A high-quality probiotic actually helps to ensure maximum absorption, thus, maximum health benefits.

The journey to health for many certainly begins with a complete blend of amino acids, because vitamins and minerals simply are not enough to address our comprehensive health needs in today's world. As the new frontiers indicate, we are only just beginning to unveil the vital applications of the amazing amino acids!

Thus, the amazing amino acids are integral to your ability to support foundational wellness and disease prevention for life!

About Dr. Daniel Smith

Dr. Daniel Smith is a former organic farmer, former advisory member for the International Organic Inspectors Association, 25-year chiropractor in Alamo, CA, and member of the California Chiropractic Association. Currently, Dr. Smith practices chiropractic part time, serves as CEO of Genesa Inc., and lectures to a variety of audiences.

In 2004, Dr. Dan became involved with organic farming by purchasing an apple orchard, a platform that provided a catalyst for research and development in collaboration with the California Certified Organic Farmers Association. As a chiropractor, Dr. Smith realized that many of his patients could be taking more responsibility for their health through diet and nutrition; a holistic approach to balanced health.

In 2006, while researching the effects of nutrition on the brain and nervous system, Dr. Smith discovered a missing link in the field, amino acids. His blend, Total Amino Solution®, quickly became an amino acid best seller after release and is now sold around the world. This wonderful response resulted in further interest and research into the effects of healthy eating and the importance of nutrition as a viable, necessary modality of integrative medicine.

In 2010, Dr. Smith began production of a video documentary, "Love of the Land." This project evolved in the Lake Tahoe area from a grass roots passion and community interest for healthy soil, healthy eating and knowledge of where one's food is coming from, including farming, delivery of healthy food to table, food to hospitals, senior citizens, and food to schools, despite local limitations.

This was the setting that provided Dr. Smith's clear vision to move forward and provide documentation. If it can be done in a mountain community, it can be done anywhere. The first film, "Love of the Land" was completed in the summer of 2011. It is Dr. Smith's vision that healthcare professionals, educators and the community at large will ultimately embrace the value that the food we eat is a significant part of our nation's new health care delivery system.

Today Dr. Smith remains focused on amino acid research as well as community nutrition because the field of application for amino acids is as vast and complex as the human body's needs for nutrients. It is this incredibly innovative, contemporary path that Dr. Smith has chosen for his professional endeavors into optimal health.

Dr. Smith's public speaking presentations include: *Micronutrients for Mental Health*, Hotel Monaco, Calif., 2009; New York Academy of Medicine, N.Y., 2011-2013, *Nutrition for the Brain and Nervous System*, 2006-12 and *Fields to Forks/ Toolbox for the Informed Eater*, Truckee, Calif. 2010-2013.

Please contact Genesa, Inc. @ 1-800-404-1065 for lecture dates or information on booking Dr. Dan as a speaker.

References

1) Shipman, J. and Wilson, J., Introduction to Physical Science, 6th Ed., D. C. Heath, 1990.

2) Maes M, Ombelet W, Verkerk R, Bosmans E, Scharpe S. Effects of pregnancy and delivery on the availability of plasma tryptophan to the brain: relationships to delivery-induced immune activation and early post-partum anxiety and depression. Psychol Med 2001 Jul;31(5):847-58.

3) Scognamiglio R, Avogaro A, Negut C, Piccolotto R, de Kreutzenberg SV, Tiengo A. The effects of oral amino acid intake on ambulatory capacity in elderly subjects. Aging ClinExp Res 2004 Dec;16(6):443-7.

4) Esmarck B, Andersen JL, Olsen S, Richter EA, Mizuno M, Kjaer M. Timing of postexercise protein intake is important for muscle hypertrophy with resistance training in elderly humans. J Physiol 2001 Aug 15;535(Pt 1):301-11.

5) Bird SP, Tarpenning KM, Marino FE. Effects of liquid carbohydrate/essential amino acid ingestion on acute hormonal response during a single bout of resistance exercise in untrained men. Nutrition 2006 Apr;22(4):367-75.

6) Ohtani M, Sugita M, Maruyama K. Amino acid mixture improves training efficiency in athletes. J Nutr 2006 Feb;136(2):538S-43S.

7) Willoughby DS, Stout JR, Wilborn CD. Effects of resistance training and protein plus amino acid supplementation

on muscle anabolism, mass & strength. Amino Acids 2006 Sep 20.

8)   Marsa M, Lozano C, Herranz A et al. Acute tryptophan depletion in eating disorders. ActasEspPsiquiatr 2006 Nov;34(6):397-402.

9)   Calder PC, Kew S. The immune system: a target for functional foods? Br J Nutr 2002 Nov;88 Suppl 2:S165-77.:S165-S177.

10) Grimble RF. Nutritional modulation of immune function. ProcNutrSoc 2001 Aug;60(3):389-97.

11) Lesch KP, Merschdorf U. Impulsivity, aggression, and serotonin: a molecular psychobiological perspective. BehavSci Law 2000;18(5):581-604.

12) Evans WJ. Protein nutrition, exercise and aging. J Am CollNutr 2004;23(6 Suppl):601S-9S.

13) Stuerenburg HJ, Stangneth B, Schoser BG. Age related profiles of free amino acids in human skeletal muscle. NeuroEndocrinolLett 2006;27(1-2):133-6.

14) Aquilani R, Viglio S, Iadarola P, Opasich C, Testa A, Dioguardi FS, Pasini E. Oral amino acid supplements improve exercise capacities in elderly patients with chronic heart failure. Am J Cardiol 2008;101(11A):104E-10E.

15) Kalantar-Zadeh K, Anker SD, Horwich TB, Fonarow GC. Nutritional and anti-inflammatory interventions in chronic heart failure. Am J Cardiol 2008;101(11A):89E-103E.

16) Pansarasa O, Flati V, Corsetti G, Brocca L, Pasini E, D'Antona G. Oral amino acid supplementation counteracts age-induced sarcopenia in elderly rats. Am J Cardiol 2008;101(11A):35E-41E.

17) Solerte SB, Gazzaruso C, Bonacasa R, Rondanelli M, Zamboni M, Basso C, Locatelli E, Schifino N, Giustina A, Fioravanti M. Nutritional supplements with oral amino

acid mixtures increases whole-body lean mass and insulin sensitivity in elderly subjects with sarcopenia. Am J Cardiol 2008;101(11A):69E-77E.

18) Fujita S, Volpi E. Amino acids and muscle loss with aging. J Nutr 2006;136(1 Suppl):277S-80S.

19) Pellegrino MA, Patrini C, Pasini E, Brocca L, Flati V, Corsetti G, D'Antona G. Amino acid supplementation counteracts metabolic and functional damage in the diabetic rat heart. Am J Cardiol 2008;101(11A):49E-56E.

20) Nisoli E, Cozzi V, Carruba MO. Amino acids and mitochondrial biogenesis. Am J Cardiol 2008;101(11A):22E-5E.

21) Brocca L, D'Antona G, Bachi A, Pellegrino MA. Amino acid supplements improve native antioxidant enzyme expression in the skeletal muscle of diabetic mice. Am J Cardiol 2008;101(11A):57E-62E.

22) Taegtmeyer H, Harinstein ME, Gheorghiade M. More than bricks and mortar: comments on protein and amino acid metabolism in the heart. Am J Cardiol 2008;101(11A):3E-7E.

23) Evans WJ. Effects of exercise on senescent muscle. ClinOrthopRelat Res 2002;(403 Suppl):S211-S220.

24) Masley SC, Weaver W, Peri G, Phillips SE. Efficacy of lifestyle changes in modifying practical markers of wellness and aging. AlternTher Health Med 2008;14(2):24-9.

25) Wagner KH, Haber P, Elmadfa I. Thanks to body exercise, getting mobile and being less dependent. Ann NutrMetab 2008;52 Suppl 1:38-42

26) Aquilani R, Viglio S, Iadarola P, Opasich C, Testa A, Dioguardi FS, Pasini E. Oral amino acid supplements improve exercise capacities in elderly patients with chronic heart failure. Am J Cardiol 2008;101(11A):104E-10E.

27) Scognamiglio R, Testa A, Aquilani R, Dioguardi FS, Pasini E. Impairment in walking capacity and myocardial function in the elderly: is there a role for nonpharmacologic therapy with nutritional amino acid supplements? Am J Cardiol 2008;101(11A):78E-81E.

28) Fillit H, Nash DT, Rundek T, Zuckerman A. Cardiovascular risk factors & dementia. Am J GeriatrPharmacother 2008;6(2):100-18.

29) Janson M. Orthomolecular medicine: the therapeutic use of dietary supplements for anti-aging. ClinInterv Aging 2006;1(3):261-5.

30) San FC, Taylor MR, Mestroni L, Botto LD, Longo N. Cardiomyopathy and carnitine deficiency. Mol Genet Metab 2008;94(2):162-6.

31) Dawson R, Jr. Taurine in aging and models of neurodegeneration. AdvExp Med Biol 2003;526:537-45.

32) Grimble RF. The effects of sulfur amino acid intake on immune function in humans. J Nutr 2006;136(6 Suppl):1660S-5S.

33) Louzada PR, Lima AC, Mendonca-Silva DL, Noel F, De Mello FG, Ferreira ST. Taurine prevents the neurotoxicity of beta-amyloid and glutamate receptor agonists: activation of GABA receptors and possible implications for Alzheimer's disease and other neurological disorders. FASEB J 2004;18(3):511-8.

34) Pierno S, De LA, Camerino C, Huxtable RJ, Camerino DC. Chronic administration of taurine to aged rats improves the electrical and contractile properties of skeletal muscle fibers. J PharmacolExpTher 1998;286(3):1183-90.

35) Takihara K, Azuma J, Awata N, Ohta H, Sawamura A, Kishimoto S, Sperelakis N. Taurine's possible protective role in age-dependent response to calcium paradox. Life Sci 1985;37(18):1705-10.

36) Taurine improves learning and retention in aged mice. NeurosciLett 2008;436(1):19-22.

37) Roth E. Immune and cell modulation by amino acids. ClinNutr 2007;26(5):535-44.

38) Ames, Bruce. A role for supplements in optimizing health: the metabolic tune-up. Archives of Biochemistry and Biophysics. 2004;423(1:227-234).

39) Eric R. Braverman, M.D with Carl C. Pfeiffer, M.D., pH.D, The Healing Nutrients Within (New Canaan, CT: Keats, 1987), p. viii.

40) McBride BW, Kelly JM Energy cost of absorption and metabolism in the ruminant tract and liver: a review J AnimSci 1990: 68(9):2997-3010

41) Auer IO. (The small intestine as an immune organ). Fortschr Med. 1990;108(15):292-296

42) Probiotics and prebiotics in dietetics practice; http://www.ncbi.nlm.nih.gov/pubmed/18313433

43) Laboratory Evaluations for Functional and Integrative Medicine; Ch 4: Amino Acids F-4.31—Blood Spot amino Acid Concentration after Oral Dosing

44) Laboratory Evaluations for Functional and Integrative Medicine; Ch 4: Amino Acids F-4.32—Representation of Daily Plasma amino Acid Levels

45) The Amino Revolution; Robert Erdmann, Ph.D; Ch 7: The Complete Blend

46) http://www.mcmanweb.com/apathy.html, McManamy, John. Apathy.

47) Association between nonspecific skeletal pain and vitamin D deficiency Heidari, B., Shirvani, J. S., Firouzjahi, A., Heidari, P., and Hajian-Tilaki, K. O. 2010 Int.J.Rheum.Dis.

48) Vitamin D deficiency: the time to ignore it has passed Haroon, M. and Regan, M. J. 2010 Int.J.Rheum.Dis.

49) Profound Vitamin D Deficiency in a Diverse Group of Women during Pregnancy Living in a Sun-Rich Environment at Latitude 32 degrees N Hamilton, S. A., McNeil, R., Hollis, B. W., Davis, D. J., Winkler, J., Cook, C., Warner, G., Bivens, B., McShane, P., and Wagner, C. L. 2010 Int.J.Endocrinol.

50) Vitamin D in health and disease: Current perspectives Zhang, R. and Naughton, D. P. 2010 Nutr.J.

51) Vitamin D supplementation in adults - guidelines Marcinowska-Suchowierska, E., Walicka, M., Talalaj, M., Horst-Sikorska, W., Ignaszak-Szczepaniak, M., and Sewerynek, E. 2010 Endokrynol.Pol.

52) Epidemiology and Phenomenology of Postpartum Mood Disorders. Flynn H. Psychiatric Annals. 2005 July;35(7):544-551.

53) O'Hara, M. W. & Swain, A. M. Rates and risk of postpartum depression-a meta-analysis. International Review of Psychiatry 1996, 8, 37-54.

54) Brent K, Barfield W, and Williams C, Prevalence of Self-Reported Postpartum Depressive Symptoms --- 17 States, 2004—2005, CDC Morbidity and Mortality Weekly Report, April 11, 2008 / 57(14);361-366.

55) Current Depression Among Adults – United States, 2006 and 2008, Revised Table Estimates, Morbidity and Mortality Weekly Report, October 1, 2010 erratum, www.cdc.gov/features/dsDepression/Revised_Table_Estimates_for_Depression_MMWR_Erratum_Feb%20 2011.pdf accessed 8/27/2012.

56) Sacher, Julia, et al., Elevated brain monoamine oxidase A binding in the early postpartum period, Arch Gen Psychiatry 2010; 67(5): 468-474.

57) Wallace, Daniel and Janice. Making Sense of Fibromyalgia. Oxford University Press, New York, 1999.

58) Starlanyl, Devin., Copeland, Mary Ellen. Fibromyalgia & Chronic Myofascial Pain Syndrome. New Harbinger Publications, Inc., Oakland, CA, 1996.

59) Cartmell, John W., Nutritional Considerations in Chronic Fatigue Syndrome. Frontier Perspectives, The Center for Frontier Sciences, Philadelphia, PA, Summer-2000.

60) Forman, Brenda., Hutson, Vivian T, RD, LD, FACHE., Piemonte, Tami A, RD, LD., Weinstein, James RD. Recruit Medicine, Department of Defense, Office of The Surgeon General, US Army, Borden Institute. 2006: 581.

61) Williams JZ. Surg Clin N Am 2003.

62) Wallace E. Br J Nurs 1994.

63) Woodward, Michael GER., Sussman, Geoff OAM., Rice, Jan., Ellis, Tal., Fazio, Virginia RDN. Expert Guide for Healthcare Professionals: Nutrition and Wound Healing.

64) Williams JZ, Barbul A. Nutrition and wound healing. Surg Clin North Am. 2003 Jun;83(3):571-96. Review.

65) Wallace E. Feeding the wound: nutrition and wound care. Br J Nurs. 1994 Jul 14-27;3(13):662-7.

66) Witte MB, Barbul A. Arginine physiology and its implication for wound healing. Wound Repair Regen. 2003 Nov-Dec;11(6):419-23. Review.

67) Children's Hospital of Philadelphia (news : web) http://www.physorg.com/news179423402.html

68) Characteristics of ADHD Disorder Among Omani Schoolchildren Using DSM-IV: Descriptive StudyJournal of Attention Disorders; January 13, 2010.

69) Pauling, Linus. "Orthomolecular Psychiatry" Science 160:265-271, 1968.

70) http://lpi.oregonstate.edu/lpbio/lpbio2.html, Linus Pauling Institute

71) Depression: prevalence, risks, and the nutrition link--a review of the literature. Leung BM, Kaplan BJ. J Am Diet Assoc. 2009 Sep;109(9):1566-75.

72) Nutritional therapies for mental disorders. Shaheen E Lakhan* and Karen F Vieira. Nutrition Journal 2008, 7:2.

73) Excess dietary methionine markedly increases the vitamin B-6 requirement of young chicks, Scherer, C. S. and Baker, D. H. 2000 J.Nutr.

74) Vitamin neurotoxicity Snodgrass, S. R. 1992 Mol. Neurobiol.

75) Is excess folic acid supplementation a risk factor for autism? Beard, C. M., Panser, L. A., and Katusic, S. K. 3-29-2011 Med.Hypotheses

76) Effects of altered maternal folic Acid, vitamin B(12) and docosahexaenoic Acid on placental global DNA methylation patterns in wistar rats Kulkarni, A., Dangat, K., Kale, A., Sable, P., Chavan-Gautam, P., and Joshi, S. 2011 PLoS.One.

77) Micronutrients prevent cancer and delay aging Ames, B. N. 12-28-1998 Toxicol.Lett.

78) High-dose vitamin therapy stimulates variant enzymes with decreased coenzyme binding affinity (increased K(m)): relevance to genetic disease and polymorphisms Ames, B. N., Elson-Schwab, I., and Silver, E. A. 2002 Am.J.Clin.Nutr.

79) http://holisticpsychiatrist.com/2009/07/14/amino-acids-key-to-comfort-for-withdrawal/. Lee, Alice. M.D.

Appendix A

How to Take Amino Acids:
Dosing, Safety and Precautions with Broad Spectrum, Free-Form Amino Acids

Relieving Relative Deficiencies

A complete blend of amino acids provides benefits without needing to measure exactly which amino acids are deficient, or, to state it another way, why "a rising tide lifts all boats." This cost effective approach, the use of a complete blend for therapeutic and daily maintenance purposes, is optimal when suggested dosages are followed.

Complete Blend Daily Serving Recommendations

Take 2,350 mg once or twice daily between meals. For optimal results or acute symptoms it may be necessary to double or triple the suggested dosage.

For wellness and prevention:
Take 2,350 mg – 4,700 mg daily.

For therapeutic effects:
Take 4,700 mg – 9,400 mg daily.

For intensive athletic performance training:
Take 4,700 mg – 9,400 mg before and after each workout.

In general, to maximize the effects of a complete blend, take the capsules on an empty stomach.

Additional Suggestions for Usage:

For more specific purposes and/or symptoms, the capsules may be taken at specific times or with beverages that enhance effectiveness. See the list below:

- Stress and anxiety conditions:
  Take capsules with water, herb tea and or vitamin C powder packs.
- Sleeplessness:
  Take with water or decaffeinated herbal tea.
- Carbohydrate cravings:
  Take with a high-grade loose green tea (natural fat burning qualities).
- Fatigue and fibromyalgia:
  Take with vitamin C powder packs to strengthen your immune system, transport the long branch chain amino acids into your skeletal muscle cells and to maximize tryptophan, tyrosine, GABA and threonine into the nervous system to balance neurotransmitters.
- Chronic back pain/recovery from surgery:
  Take with vitamin C powder packs. Vitamin C and amino acids are the building blocks for collagen. This combination

of vitamin C and amino acids offers the building blocks to restore tissue injury.

- Wellness and prevention:
Take with water, herbal tea, vitamin C powder packs, or a super-fruit juice.
- Athletic performance:
Take with a high-quality electrolyte mix.

Precautions Using Broad Spectrum Amino Acid Supplements

1. Dose varies from individual to individual.
2. When taking medications along with a complete blend, always consult your physician.
3. Be alert for possible kidney or liver problems.
4. With stomach ulcer; note that amino acids can be slightly acidic.
5. If you are pregnant or nursing, consult your physician.
6. If you have had previous reactions to supplements, foods, or medications with unusual or uncomfortable symptoms, consult your physician.
7. If you are suffering from a serious physical illness, particularly cancer, consult your physician.
8. If you have a genetic deficit, consult your physician.
9. If discomfort of any kind is experienced when taking any supplement, stop taking and re-evaluate.

DISCLAIMER

You should consult your physician or other health care professional before starting any supplement to determine if it is right for your needs. You should not rely on this information as a substitute for, nor does it replace, professional medical advice, diagnosis, or treatment. If you have any concerns or questions about your health, you should always consult with a physician or other health-care professional.

Do not disregard, avoid or delay obtaining medical or health related advice from your health-care professional because of something you may have read in this book. The use of any information provided here is solely at your own risk.

Future developments in medical research may impact the health, fitness and nutritional advice that appear here. No assurance can be given that the advice contained here will always include the most recent findings or developments with respect to the particular material.

Appendix B

Amino Detoxification

There are many reasons our body's innate ability to form neurotransmitters has been compromised. Some of the most common reasons include poor dietary intake, addiction to harmful substances, environmental toxins, disease and/or a family history of mental illness.

This can lead to symptoms of depression, anxiety, lack of focus, insomnia, weight gain, and increased addiction. However, amino acids supplementation can often re-establish proper levels of circulating neurotransmitters, thus mitigating both the recurrence of symptoms as well as possible withdrawal effects. This can be accomplished many times through a simple process of standard amino detoxification. Other benefits and types of amino detoxification:

- Improved mental clarity and acuity: "Refocus Detox"
- A sense of being recharged: "Recharge Detox"
- Contribution to overall wellness and prevention: "Optimal Detox"

You will want to start slowly with an amino detoxification as too much toxic released in your system too quickly will backfire and cause you enough discomfort to consider stopping the program.

Week One: Loading Phase

---

1. Take 2,350 mg 4 times per day. Take them first thing in the morning, midmorning, midafternoon and before bedtime.
2. Take two high-quality, chelated vitamin/mineral supplements two times per day, once at breakfast and once at lunch. It is essential the vitamin/mineral formula meet certain guidelines including formulation with chelated minerals. The chelated minerals allow the ingredients to pass through your stomach wall to get into all the cells of your body, including passing through the brain blood barrier to get deep into all the cells that are starving for these essential minerals for healthy brain function.
3. Take 1,000 mg of sodium ascorbate four times per day.
4. Find a certified therapist in your region. Regular therapy sessions during this detoxification and healing phase will give you the best chance for a successful outcome.

Week Two: Loading Phase *continued*

---

1. Take 2,350 mg four times per day. Take them first thing in the morning, midmorning, midafternoon and/or before bedtime.
2. Take two high-quality, chelated mineral supplements two times per day, once at breakfast and once at lunch.

3. Take 1,000 mg of sodium ascorbate four times per day.
4. Continue with one to two therapy sessions per week.

After week two you will have completed the loading dose. Your body's cells are now almost completely filled with all the essential nutrients required for optimal health. The chemicals that were toxic to your system are now being flushed out!

Week Three through Six: Healing Phase

1. Take 2,350 mg 3 times per day. Take them first thing in the morning, midmorning & midafternoon or before bedtime.
2. Take two high-quality, chelated vitamin/mineral supplements two times per day, once at breakfast and once at lunch.
3. Take 1,000 mg of sodium ascorbate four times per day.
4. Continue with one to two sessions of therapy per week.
5. Include time in a sauna or steam room.

To continue the detoxification process during the healing phase, it is important to find a hot sauna, infrared sauna and/or a steam room. It is best to go into the sauna or steam room as close to daily as possible during the healing phase. The sweating allows for the body to release toxic chemicals that get stored in the fat cells and the liver cells.

It has been shown that some prescription drugs can remain in cells for years after you stop taking them. If you do the sweats, try to stay in the room for 15 to 45 minutes for maximum benefits. If you have a history of high blood pressure, you need to check with your medical doctor before doing this phase of the recovery.

Week Seven: Wellness Phase

At this point in the healing cycle, you should be feeling fairly stable and able to maintain quality eating habits of three healthy meals and four to eight glasses of water per day. The amino acid and supplement routine has now done the powerful work they are designed to do—detoxify, repair, heal and balance. It is important that you maintain some level of intake of all three supplements to maintain your progress.

Maintenance

I recommend you add into your daily supplement intake a good probiotic for gastrointestinal health and omega 3 fish oil. Each of these recommendations will assure that your body is receiving all the essential micronutrients and probiotics it requires to maintain optimal health and wellness.

Of course, healthy eating is a must! All these supplements work hand in hand with good, healthy food. And, last but not least, I strongly recommend that you continue therapy sessions two times per month for one to three months to fully integrate and support your new lifestyle.

NOTE: If you've had a history of any autoimmune disorders, such as liver, kidney, spleen, or heart disease you should discuss the integration of any detox program with your healthcare professional prior to beginning.

Appendix C

Vegetarians and Free-Form Amino Acid Supplementation

It is particularly challenging to get all the essential amino acids in every meal as a vegetarian. During my design of a complete amino acid blend I intentionally included vegetarian and vegan requirements including encapsulating the blend in a vegi-capsule to assure all vegetarian standards had been met. A typical vegetarian/vegan diet poses nutritional challenges and makes it difficult to achieve optimum health. For example, people on a vegan diet may have difficulty consuming enough protein, vitamin B12, and vitamin D.

When contemplating protein alternatives to meat, understand that food items lacking essential amino acids are poor sources of protein equivalents. A balanced protein source including every single one of the essential amino acids supported by many nonessential amino acids is necessary for a high degree of *net protein utilization*, which is the fraction of amino acids converted to proteins from the amino acids supplied.

Did you know that scientists have determined the chicken egg to be nature's most biologically complete protein for human consumption? How can a vegetarian or vegan mimic the protein of an egg without actually eating an egg? Perhaps there's a way.

What we know about proteins: Complete proteins contain a balanced set of essential amino acids for humans. Animal sources such as meat, poultry, eggs, fish, milk, and cheese provide all of those essential amino acids. However, if you're a vegetarian or vegan, you can find near-complete proteins in some plant sources such as quinoa, buckwheat, hempseed and amaranth, among others. A popular alternative protein source is soy, but soy is lower in sulfur-containing amino acids (methionine and cysteine), which instead are abundant in other plant protein sources. The good news for vegetarians and vegans is that it's not necessary to consume plant foods containing complete proteins as long as a reasonably varied diet of near complete proteins is maintained. This can be accomplished by consuming a wide variety of plant foods where a full set of essential amino acids are supplied and the human body can convert the amino acids into proteins.

According to Jack Norris, R.D., in *The Vegan Society and Vegan Outreach*, there are no reliable unfortified plant sources of vitamin B12; therefore, fortified foods and/or supplements are necessary for the optimal health of vegans. Deficiencies in vitamin B12 can have serious health consequences, including anemia and neurodegenerative disorders. A complete blend can address both the concern with a variety of protein sources as well as providing necessary B12 for vegetarians and vegans. Being educated about appropriate choices for optimal dietary intake is the necessary component to designing a successful vegetarian or vegan diet.

Appendix D

Figures and Images

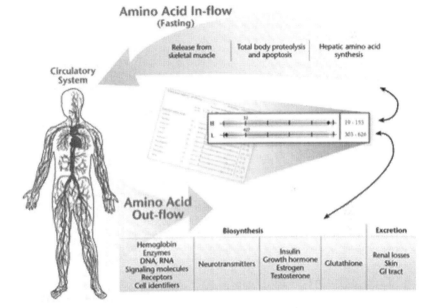

Figure 4.2 — Sources and Destinations of Plasma Amino Acids

The amount of amino acids in the free form in plasma is very small compared with plasma protein concentrations. In humans, biosynthesis cannot yield EAA and in the fasting state portal supply is absent. Concentrations of EAA measured in fasting plasma, therefore, are determined by the flux into the blood from tissue protein degradation balanced with flux out of the blood for protein synthesis, excretion, oxidation and formation of non-protein products.

Figure 4.2

Lord RS, Bralley JA, eds. Laboratory Evaluations for Integrative and Functional Medicine. Duluth, GA: Metametrix Institute; 2008.

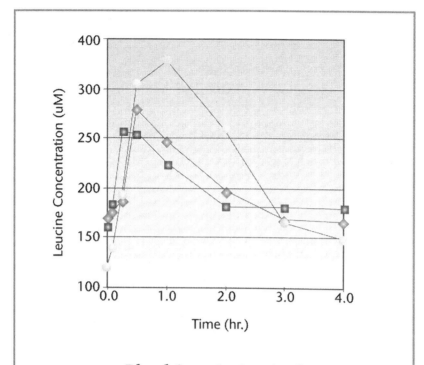

FIGURE 4.31 — **Blood Spot Amino Acid Concentrations after Oral Dosing**

Three healthy adult fasting males submitted blood spot specimens at the intervals shown after consuming a 10 g bolus of free-form amino acids containing 1.3 g of L-leucine. The three different symbols show an individual subject's results from the eight dried blood spot specimens collected over the 4-hour interval. Leucine concentrations were determined by quantitative LC-MS/MS analysis.

Figure 4.31

Lord RS, Bralley JA, eds. Laboratory Evaluations for Integrative and Functional Medicine. Duluth, GA: Metametrix Institute; 2008.

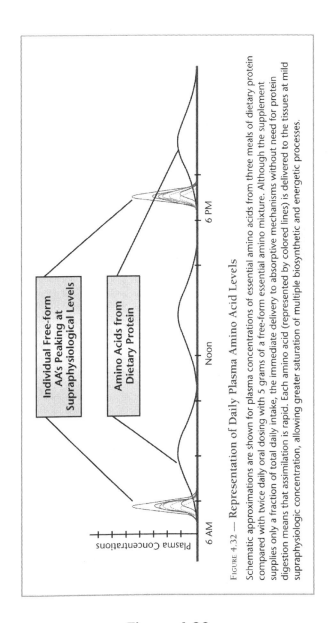

FIGURE 4.32 — Representation of Daily Plasma Amino Acid Levels

Schematic approximations are shown for plasma concentrations of essential amino acids from three meals of dietary protein compared with twice daily oral dosing with 5 grams of a free-form essential amino mixture. Although the supplement supplies only a fraction of total daily intake, the immediate delivery to absorptive mechanisms without need for protein digestion means that assimilation is rapid. Each amino acid (represented by colored lines) is delivered to the tissues at mild supraphysiologic concentration, allowing greater saturation of multiple biosynthetic and energetic processes.

Figure 4.32

Lord RS, Bralley JA, eds. Laboratory Evaluations for Integrative and Functional Medicine. Duluth, GA: Metametrix Institute; 2008.

Made in the USA
San Bernardino, CA
21 May 2018